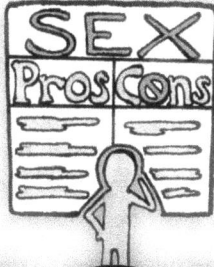

The Teen Guide to Sex

WITHOUT REGRETS

By Youth Communication

Written and edited by
the teen writers at Youth Communication,
and Andrea Estepa, Keith Hefner,
Laura Longhine, Rachel Blustain, and Nora McCarthy

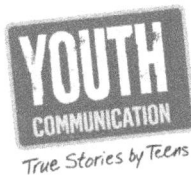

True Stories by Teens

The Teen Guide to Sex
(WITHOUT REGRETS)

EXECUTIVE EDITORS
Keith Hefner and Laura Longhine

CONTRIBUTING EDITORS
Clarence Haynes, Andrea Estepa, Kendra Hurley,
Nora McCarthy, Tamar Rothenberg, Rachel Blustain,
Philip Kay and Al Desetta

LAYOUT & DESIGN
Efrain Reyes, Jr.

COVER
YC Art Dept.

ILLUSTRATOR
Gamal Jones

For reprint information, please contact Youth Communication.

ISBN 978-1-935552-28-4

Printed in the United States of America

Youth Communication ®
New York, New York
www.youthcomm.org

Catalog Item #YD-SEX

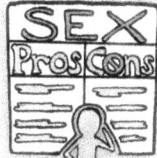

The

Teen
Guide
to
Sex

WITHOUT REGRETS

Table of Contents

Chapter 3

Chapter 4

Chapter 5

Chapter 6

Chapter 7

Chapter 8

WHAT TO EXPECT: TEENS SHARE THEIR EXPERIENCES

Chapter 9

THE MORNING AFTER: TEENS SHARE THEIR EXPERIENCES

Practical Info

About Us

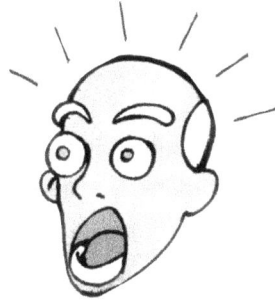

Chapter 1

Ten Things to Ask About Yourself

Have you made a *decision* that you want to have sex?

A lot of teenagers say that their first sexual experience wasn't something they planned. Instead, it "just happened." While being spontaneous and going with the flow can be fun, it can also lead to regret. That's because sex comes with emotional and physical risks, like heartbreak, pregnancy, and STDs (sexually transmitted diseases).

If you plan ahead you can reduce these risks, and make sex safer and more enjoyable. That means figuring out what you want from a sexual relationship and choosing a partner who is looking for the same things. It also means deciding what kind of protection you're going to use and having it handy. If you don't plan, pregnancy and STDs can also "just happen."

You're more likely to do the things you need to do to prepare for sex (like discussing it with your partner and getting protection) if you've admitted to yourself that you want to have sex. This can be harder than it sounds. For example, it may be particularly difficult for girls who have been raised to believe that they shouldn't have the same kind of power-

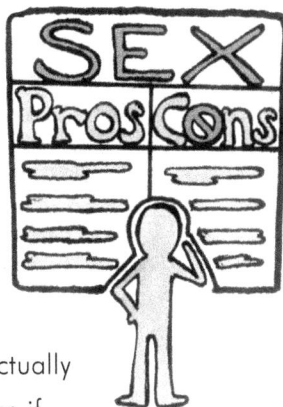

ful sexual feelings that guys do. Girls
and guys who have been taught they
should wait until marriage may convince themselves that they're not going
to have sex—until the moment they're actually
doing it! It can also be hard for gay teens if
they've been taught that their feelings are wrong
or not normal.

However, if you don't realize or admit that you might act
on your sexual feelings, then sex—and all the related things
that could happen—are much more likely to "just happen"
to you.

Of course, you can decide that you're physically and emotionally ready to have sex but still wait weeks, months, or
even years before actually having sex. And you have the
right to change your mind. *Whether* you have sex is not as
important as being thoughtful and reflective, so that you
make the choice that's right for *you*.

Are you planning to wait until marriage?

You may choose to abstain from sex until marriage, or until you're much older, because of your values or religion. Don't let anyone make you feel weird or self-conscious about sticking to those values. If someone tells you that "everyone" has sex before marriage, remember that that's just not true. One recent study found that more half of the teens surveyed were still virgins at the time they graduated from high school.

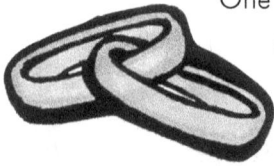

What would your parents say?

Some teens find that their parents are supportive and welcome their questions about sex. But if you think your parents would be deeply disappointed or stop trusting you if they found out you were having sex, that's one factor to consider. Would they kick you out of the house and tell you they never wanted to speak to you again? What if it meant that they'd also be finding out that you're gay? Or pregnant? Or have an STD? If you're pretty sure that having sex would hurt your relationship with your parents, you need to consider that.

Don't just assume you can keep it a secret. You may not be able to.

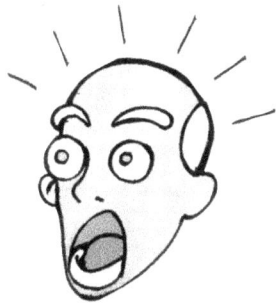

Do you know why you want to have sex?

This may seem like a silly question, but if you don't know why you want to have sex, chances are you'll wind up feeling disappointed when you do. There are lots of good reasons to have sex, including that you love each other and that you both want to take that step.

But there are also lots of reasons that teens (and adults!) have sex that make them look back and think, "Boy, that was a dumb thing to do." Some of those reasons include:

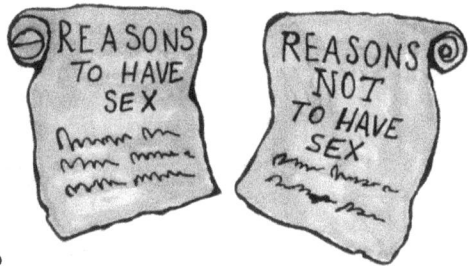

- To please someone else, even though you don't want to
- To make someone jealous
- To feel more mature (Having sex when you're not ready will probably make you feel crummy, not more mature.)

- Because you're being pressured
- Because everyone else is doing it (They're not, and besides, you're not everyone else.)
- To make someone more loyal to you (It's unlikely.)
- To feel better about yourself (It usually doesn't work.)
- Because you want to say you had sex with that person
- Because you heard sex is good
- To get it over with

Before having sex, think about your motivation (your reasons). Don't just ask yourself if you want to do it. Ask *why* you want to do it. Make sure having sex is something you want to do for yourself, not because you're trying to impress or please or change someone else, or because you have something to prove.

Do you know which gender you're attracted to?

Don't laugh. Although most people know from early child-hood whether they're attracted to the same sex or the opposite sex and never waver, not everyone is so sure (or so consistent). Sometimes teens who have always thought they were heterosexual will develop a crush on a friend or teach-er of the same sex and wonder if that means they're really gay. Sometimes kids who have homosexual feelings will try to convince themselves that they're not gay, because it's not accepted in their family, culture, or religion.

Some people are bisexual. That means they are sincerely attracted to both men and women. Others may identify as transgender. If you do, it is very likely that you feel attracted to people of the same sex. What's different about being transgender is that you feel as though you were born into the wrong body—that you're really of the opposite sex.

And lastly, some people find that who they're attracted to changes over time.

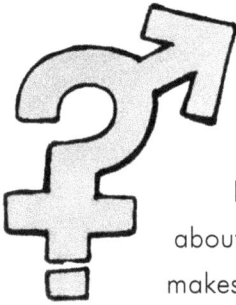

So how do you figure out whether you really want to have sex with a guy or a girl? Listen to your body, your heart, and your imagination. Forget about what other people might say. Who makes your heart beat faster or gets you tingling? Who do you want to kiss? Who have you dated in the past? Did you really enjoy being with that person or were you just going through the motions? Who do you fantasize about? (If you masturbate, who do you think about while you do it?)

You may have to experiment a little before you can be sure. Give yourself a chance to find out who you really want to be with.

Do you feel attractive?

Hardly anyone is completely happy with the way they look. Too fat, too thin, too tall, too short, too light, too dark, too big, not big enough.

What does this have to do with sex? A lot.

If you don't think that you're very good-looking, it may be hard to imagine someone wanting to have sex with you. And that can make you want to go out and have sex just to prove to yourself that somebody wants you. Unfortunately, just because someone wants to have sex with you, doesn't mean they want *you*. And if you're already feeling insecure, having sex with someone who doesn't want to have anything more to do with you afterwards isn't going to make you feel better about yourself. It will probably make you feel worse.

If you think you're not attractive and never will be, that's probably not true. Most people take time to grow comfortable with their body and their sexuality.

And if you think no one is ever going to want to have sex with you because you're not good-looking enough, look around. You'll see plenty of folks who will never make *People*'s list of the "50 Most Beautiful" holding hands and making out. (And look at all those less-than-gorgeous adults pushing baby carriages.)

The thing you need to remember is: you don't have to look like a movie star for another human being to find you attractive and want to be with you. The old saying is true—beauty *is* in the eye of the beholder. And someone who finds you attractive is going to make you feel attractive—because of the way they look at you and talk to you and touch you.

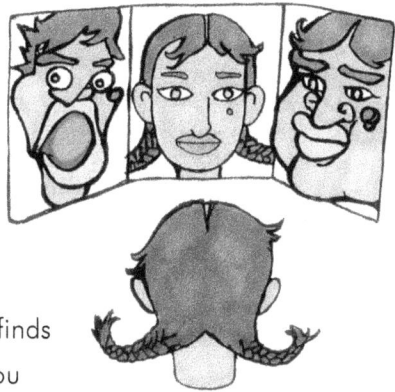

If you're thinking about having sex with someone who doesn't make you feel attractive, who makes you more self-conscious about your looks rather than less, think again. You can do better.

Are you ready to behave responsibly?

What does it mean to be responsible? There's no easy answer to that question, but here's a general rule: being responsible means that if you decide to have sex, you take that decision seriously. That means that you take necessary precautions against pregnancy and disease, and are honest, thoughtful, caring, and respectful of your partner—whether you're in a long-term relationship or just together for a night.

For example, a girl who tells a guy she's having sex with that she's on the pill when she isn't is not being responsible; neither is a guy who refuses to use a condom because "sex feels better without it." It means you have the self-control *not* to do something you will feel guilty about—like having sex with your friend's guy or girl. It also means that you talk *before* you have sex about what you would do if you (or your girlfriend) gets pregnant.

Have you said "no"
when you wanted to?

If someone asks you to do something that makes you uncomfortable—like fool around when your parents are home or have oral sex when you're not sure how you feel about it—you should be able to tell that person you don't want to. If you agree to do something and then change your mind—even after you've started messing around—you should be able to stop without worrying that the other person is going to get angry or abusive. And if someone touches you in a way that hurts or feels wrong or just doesn't make you feel excited, you should feel comfortable asking that person to stop or to do something different.

Being able to say "no" whenever you want to is important. Saying no can be hard, which is why it's good to practice standing up for yourself before it ever comes to sex. Saying no when you don't want to do something shows that you respect yourself and know how to take care of yourself.

How well do you know yourself?

Have you ever had the experience of a parent, a friend (or even an enemy) telling you something about yourself that you thought showed amazing, brilliant insight into who you are? Then you excitedly mentioned this insight to another friend, and she said, "Of course, I knew that about you all along."

The fact is, there is a lot we don't know about ourselves. We're just too deep inside who we are to always be able to see ourselves clearly.

So what does that have to do with sex? A lot. Wanting to have sex at a particular time or with a particular person is motivated by all kinds of desires, some of which you are not even aware of. Say your father's never been there for you. You might be attracted to an older guy who promises he always will be. Or maybe you get upset easily. You might find yourself attracted to someone who's in control when you feel out of control. Maybe you didn't get the kind of emotional support you needed at home. As a result, you might feel too afraid to open up, and might rather just have sex without the emotional relationship.

Because so much of who you are goes into your sexual feelings, it helps to think through what you want from your romantic and sexual relationships, and why. It's also a good idea to talk to family members or friends who know you well. Understanding yourself better might not change who you're attracted to, but it can help you make better decisions about what to do when you feel that rush of attraction.

Have you talked to someone you trust about whether you're ready for sex?

You're the only one who can figure out whether or not you're ready. But talking it over with someone you trust can really help. It could be a parent, an older sibling, a favorite aunt or uncle, a friend of the family, a counselor, or your best friend. Choose someone who will listen and help you sort out your feelings, someone you can be honest with about your fears or questions, someone who can help you figure out the ways that having sex will affect your life, both

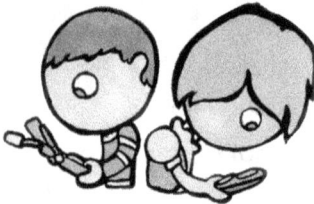

physically and emotionally.

Whenever you have to make an important decision, it's good to think ahead to both the positive and negative things that could happen as a result. Talking with someone who knows you well about the pros and cons of sex can make it easier to figure out what you really want to do. Sometimes just saying out loud what's been running through your mind can help you better understand your feelings.

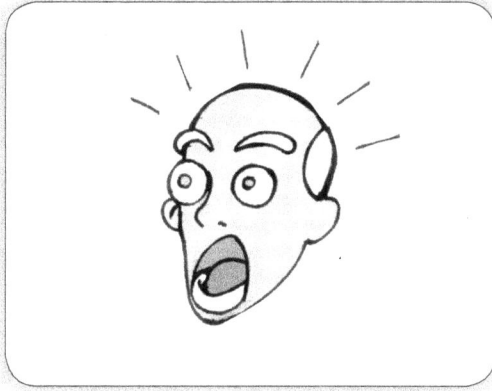

Am I Ready to Have Sex?

Teens Share Their Experiences

Womanhood Can Wait

By Nicole Hawkins

Sometimes when I'm walking down the block I'll see a 12-year-old girl with hardly any clothes on, and I'll wonder if this little girl knows something more than I know. What inside of her makes her want to possess and advertise such sexuality when it is too much for me to deal with?

I am 18 years old, but I'm not exactly sure if I'm an 18-year-old woman or an 18-year-old girl. Lots of times I feel like I'm on my way. But other times I feel clueless, like everything is still new and a mystery to me. It seems like girls are always in a hurry to grow up and become women — and part of being a woman means having boyfriends and having sex. But I'm still struggling to understand who I am, and I'm not sure I'm ready for womanhood yet.

At a young age I was taught that boys were bad while girls were nice and made up of sugar and spice. I was told to defend myself against boys any way I knew how, including scratching their eyeballs out. I was told that if I had sex before I got married, I would be disowned and put in a home. Maybe my father felt that since he waited until he was about 22 years old to have sex with my mother, I, a female, should have no problem holding out. My mother was even worse. If I had sex before marriage, I would not only be considered a disappointment, but worst of all, a SLUT!

Despite these lectures, I was still very close to my father. He would say things like, "You have to do well in school so that you can be accepted into a good college, so you can be your own woman and won't have to depend on a man," and I believed him.

At the same time, he made me feel like it was OK to be a kid. Even after I started dating, my father still bought me Barbie dolls and other kid stuff. I remember feeling happy, relieved—and confused. While I was facing the idea that sooner or later I had to grow up, here was my daddy telling me, "It's OK to be a kid for as long as you can."

When I was 8 years old, my 11-year-old sister, Tamika, started puberty. Growing up was supposed to mean taking responsibility for yourself and your actions. Instead I watched my sister's body and emotions control her. The acne, PMS, cramps, awkwardness, boobs, and BOYS. Everything seemed like a tailspin. I watched my sister get hurt, either dumped or cheated on, and it made me glad that my turn was ages away. What a joy, I thought, to be able to lie on my stomach and be comfortable because my chest was completely flat.

Still, all around me people were maturing. By junior high school, the rest of my peers seemed to be well into their third or fourth relationship. I felt like something was wrong with me, unnatural. I felt like it was my duty to act mature, so I went a little boy-crazy myself. Around that time, my mother found in my diary that I had kissed a boy. When she called me a slut and a harlot, that made me want to go boy-crazy even more. Until something stopped me dead in my tracks.

I have all the time in the world to experience sex. I figure why not wait a while and experience my virginity.

My friend Sharnette and I used to hang out and get ourselves into these fine little messes. When we were 13, Sharnette started dating this guy Ricky. Ricky had a friend, Edgar, who wanted to get hooked up with me. Edgar was cute and four years older than I was. So Sharnette and I visited the boys at Ricky's house.

Edgar and I sat on the bed and talked and played video games. Then we started to kiss. Soon Edgar began to massage my breasts. Immediately I wanted to put an end to the situation, but before I could act he was pulling the ends of my shirt out of my pants. I began to panic. I stood up in a rush and proclaimed that I was leaving.

Later I found out that Edgar was planning to have sex with me that evening. After that, I became fearful of guys and all my parents' warnings raced through my head. I started to see guys as the unpredictable, conniving creatures my father described. I still wanted to explore my sexuality, but I didn't feel safe anymore.

I watched my sister get hurt, either dumped or cheated on, and it made me glad that my turn was ages away.

By the time high school started, I was also feeling more self-conscious about my body. The summer before high school, I grew a few inches and my chest swelled up to a C cup. While lots of teenage girls like attention from the opposite sex, I didn't. I hated when guys would stare at my chest and look to see if I had a nice ass. I wore baggy jeans and plaid shirts big enough to hide the protruding obstacles settled in my bra.

I became extremely shy around everyone, especially boys. For the first couple of years of high school, I don't think I ever said a full sentence. Even though I was having a really hard time, I also did a lot of growing. Being alone so much gave me space and time to explore who I was and would ultimately become.

When I was around 14 and 15, I began to question my father's beliefs. I'd tell him that I didn't know if I could wait until I got married to have sex. He thought I was in a rebellious, disrespectful stage. He was partially right, but not fully. I also really wanted answers about sex.

I started reading a lot of women's magazines. On the radio I discovered a talk show on sex and love. I would tune in every Monday through Thursday and listen to discussions about topics such as homosexuality, AIDS, cheating, virginity, femininity, even different sexual positions.

Over the next couple of years, I began to gain control of my life. My schoolwork improved. I became very spiritual for a while, and I felt like I was rediscovering myself. I also began to feel that the sexuality that was sprouting in me was natural and shouldn't be looked upon as evil.

Last fall, I entered an alternative school and soared academically. I even joined the school newspaper. I was really confident and proud of myself. I also had a job.

By finding stability in other areas of my life, I was able to begin to feel comfortable about my body and my sexuality. For the first time in a long time I felt comfortable enough to allow myself to be emotionally vulnerable. I was ready to take on the responsibility of relationships. Soon I developed friendships with males and I no longer felt threatened. After my 18th birthday, my pants also began to get tighter, my shirts smaller.

I started dating my current boyfriend a week after Valentine's Day. Even before we started dating, we were friends. We would listen to each other and make each other laugh. And after we began going out, it was incredible. For the first time in my life I actually trusted a guy almost 100%. That was something I never thought I would do.

We have a good physical relationship and we talk openly about everything we do, but I'm not ready for sex. Right now I'm still in the process of becoming a woman and growing comfortable with my sexuality.

There are times these days when I'll put on a dress and suddenly I'll feel more powerful. Occasionally you'll see me walking down the street, strutting with such self-confidence you wouldn't even recognize me. Sometimes dressing feminine can do that to a person.

Still, I often question the pros and cons of exhibiting my femininity. It seems like it could make me more powerful, more me. But I also worry if it will make me more passive, and more likely to rely on beauty to get by.

> **I began to feel that the sexuality that was sprouting in me was natural and shouldn't be looked upon as evil.**

Sometimes I'll look at the professionally dressed women on their way to work and I'll wonder whether they're as confused about themselves and life as I am. What if they're just putting on a show to make their colleagues, families, and friends believe they are Woman?

I used to believe that after your teens you get it all down pat. But as I approach adulthood, I don't find that to be true at all.

I'm glad that I've waited and not rushed into sex, because I haven't found myself yet. I'm not at the place I want to be. I have all the time in the world to experience sex. I figure why not wait a while and experience my virginity. I still have a lot to figure out.

If you asked me right now "What do you consider yourself to be?" I'd answer: a bystander, a sort of misfit, searching for my place. I'm in the midst of development. I'm like a butterfly emerging from her cocoon. I hope my metamorphosis will be a revolution.

Nicole was 18 when she wrote this story.

I Need a Girl

Being with Keesha helped me accept that I'm a lesbian

By Destiny

I was a 13-year-old high school freshman when I realized that I was attracted to females. I didn't want to face that I was seriously looking at girls like a guy would. I felt funny because I didn't know anyone who was a lesbian. I didn't understand why I was feeling this way.

I didn't think I could reveal my attractions to any of my friends, because, for us, it was about how to get boys to like you. I'd had "boyfriends," and had even kissed a boy. So I convinced myself that I was merely curious about being with the same sex.

But one girl brought a major change to how I looked at my sexuality. She lived near my house. I usually saw her around, often by the neighborhood church. But I didn't know her name. Every time I saw her, I stared and got nervous and clumsy. My heart beat like a drum, and my chest got tight. I even tripped on the curb once while watching her walk.

One day, I was with my friend Susan and we saw her again.

"Hi, Keesha," Susan said.

"Wassup, girl," Keesha replied. Susan introduced me to Keesha, and we said right there that we should hang out since we saw each other so often.

I started to spend a lot of time with Keesha on the weekends and saw her after school sometimes. We were the same age and both liked to watch horror movies and write. Sometimes we acted out our stories at home. And when we went shopping together, we bought each other gifts.

Spending time with Keesha made me like her a lot more. About two months after we were introduced, I decided to tell her how I felt about her. I knew it was risky, but I was scared that my feelings for her would get too intense if I continued to hold them in.

We were at her house one day, and I knew I had to tell her then and there. My palms were sweating and my head started to itch. Keesha had accepted that her mother's bisexual and that her best friend, Michael, is gay. Still, I didn't know how she felt about a girl having feelings for her.

So, as we were gossiping, I came out and said, "I have to tell you something."

"What?" she replied.

I stalled, and then said, "Well, before I met you, I used to see you all the time."

"You used to look at me mad funny," she said.

"Well...I was just looking because I was attracted to you," I said timidly.

Keesha looked very surprised. Then she blushed. "Well," she said. "I like you too."

This could not be real. I kept on asking her if she was serious. Although she kept saying yes, it didn't hit me until she kissed me on my lips. I'd never kissed a girl before. When I'd kissed a boy, I felt nothing. When I kissed Keesha, I felt butterflies in my stomach. Her lips felt like rose petals and tasted like orange lip-gloss.

After we got over the initial shock of our attraction to each other, Keesha and I became a couple. But we never showed it in public; we always made sure that whoever saw us thought of us as friends. We weren't ready to be criticized by other people, so we told no one about our romance.

What mattered more to me was that Keesha was in my life. I hugged her tight every time we met. I wrote her letters almost every day. We spent hours talking to each other on the phone and instant messaging each other on the computer. About a month and a half into our relationship, she told me she loved me. And I loved her too.

Unfortunately, I grew busy with dance and she with theater, and we stopped having time for each other. One night on the phone after we'd been going out about three months, I told Keesha we were drifting apart. I said we should just be friends.

She sounded sad. I felt sad too. I cried after I hung up. It was hard, but I felt it was for the best. Thankfully, we're still friends. Soon after being with her, I made up my mind that I was a lesbian, and that I didn't want to be with guys anymore. The strong love and attraction I felt for Keesha was what I knew I could feel for another girl, not a guy.

I convinced myself that I was merely curious about being with the same sex.

Three months after breaking up with Keesha, I felt comfortable enough with my sexuality to risk coming out and telling some of my friends I was a lesbian. I also told my parents. I'm 16 now, and have dated other girls since Keesha. Some of those relationships have been even better than when I dated Keesha because they were out in the open.

I have a girlfriend now. I can hold her hand in public and not care about the eyes that I know are looking at us. I can kiss her in public without looking over my shoulder to check if I see anyone I know.

My relationship with Keesha helped me get to this point. She was my first girlfriend, and I'll never forget her.

Destiny was 16 when she wrote this story.
She later graduated from high school and went on to college.

Why I Hate Sex

By Lenny Jones

Sex isn't all it's cracked up to be. Maybe I'm the only one who feels this way, but I have good reason to. I can honestly say that I am the king of reckless relationships.

When I was younger, relationships didn't really matter that much. If I found a girl attractive, I'd write her a little note or something. If she rejected me, who cared? I'd just go home and watch cartoons or play in the park with my friends.

In middle school, the pressure started to build to have a girl. All my friends did and it wasn't much fun hanging out with them and their girls. I felt like excess baggage. When I made plans to go out to the movies with a friend and he invited his girlfriend, I felt like a tag-along. It seemed like, whenever I tried to talk to my friend, he would be so preoccupied with his girl that if I walked away, he wouldn't even know I was gone. So I went hunting and found myself a girlfriend of my own.

Our relationship was one of those cute puppy love things. We were inseparable—wherever you saw one, you saw the other. We were always kissing and hugging, talking about whatever was on our minds, and just having fun making each other happy. We would set a time when we would both ask our teachers if we could go to the bathroom and we would meet by the stairs. Then we would run down the halls together and cause trouble. (What do you expect, we were only 11 or 12.) We would write little love poems and notes, then stick them into each other's lockers. I found the joy that all my friends were raving about. It actually made me want to go to school the next day so I could start it all over again.

But then my friends started having sex and telling me every intimate detail—every day! I was still a virgin and felt pretty left out again. Whenever my friends asked if I had done it yet, I would lie and say, "Yeah, I lost it!" and deflect the attention back to them. But one time I got caught out there when a friend asked me if I was still a virgin, and I said no. He kept asking me questions about things I didn't know about and couldn't answer, so I ended up getting busted. I decided to jump on the bandwagon and have sex.

I thought sex would totally transform me. People told me that it would "make your voice go deep," "put hair on your chest," "clear up acne," "make you more mature" and "make you a man." But at the same time, I was petrified of sex. People told me horror stories about it, too. A friend of a friend had a doctor put a tube where no tube should go because he had contracted an STD. I would cross my legs just thinking about that; it scared the bejeezus out of me. So did HIV/AIDS. I kept thinking about all the things that could go wrong, like condom breakage and pregnancy. But eventually, I had sex anyway.

Unfortunately, my first experience was nothing worth raving about. It wasn't really something that I wanted. Yes, I was curious. But mainly I was taken in by all the hype and I wanted to be accepted. Afterwards, I was just sitting there thinking to myself, "That's it? I want a refund!"

I started to feel betrayed by everyone who had hyped up sex.

I was so petrified that something might have gone wrong that I went for a checkup at a teen clinic the next day. They tested me for STDs and gave me a whole bunch of stuff to make sex safer, like KY jelly, flavored dental dams, some foamy stuff, and lots of condoms.

Even after that, I was still paranoid. I was taking HIV tests every month for about four months. I was also thinking about becoming a monk or celibate and taking medication to lower or stop my sperm production. I was a nut!

After a while, I started to feel betrayed by everyone who had hyped up sex. It was like an evil cycle they just had to pass down to me. They lost their virginity, regretted it, and then made it seem like the greatest thing on earth so they could get other people to share their misery.

I say that because for me, losing my virginity was like opening a bag of potato chips—it's hard to eat just one. Sex became a weird craving, both physically and emotionally. I craved it physically because of all that biological crap that goes on in a man's body. (I don't think I need to get more explicit.) I craved it emotionally (and still do) because I wanted to experience love with someone I really cared about and felt an emotional bond with.

Even though I lost my virginity several years ago, I still haven't found "Ms. Right"—only "Ms. OK" and "Ms. One Night Stand." But I really want more than just the physical side of sex. I want to experience the emotional side, too. I want to find the "right" person (if there is such a thing). Without that emotional bond, sex still feels the same way it felt the first time—boring.

That's mainly why I hate sex. It never puts my mind to rest, only my hormones. And it leaves me an emotional wreck because having sex with someone I don't really care about makes me yearn for the right person even more.

Lenny was 19 when he wrote this story.
He later worked as a researcher for travel guidebooks.

Looking for Love

By Fetima P.

My boyfriend had always known about my past, but one day toward the beginning of our relationship, he asked me how many guys I'd had sex with. "A lot," I said. But he wanted a specific number. I was shocked when I counted and realized the answer was 21. That even shocked him. So then I asked him the same question, and when he answered, I was speechless for the first time in my life. He said, "One."

I don't think I ever felt so bad in my life. Not even when people had called me names did I ever feel that bad. When I came out of shock, I burst into tears. He told me I shouldn't be upset—I really am a nice girl who didn't know what she wanted from a man, he said. Actually, I did know what I wanted from a man—the problem was, I didn't know how to get it. I wanted someone who would give me all the love and support I didn't get at home. What I got instead was just sex.

I guess I figured that if I could find a nice guy to treat me right, he would automatically take the place of my father, who left home when I was in the 6th grade. I was very hurt when my father left because we had such a good relationship. We would go to Florida by ourselves for the weekend and leave my mother home. We'd go out to dinner and to the movies. And it meant a lot to me that (and this may sound silly) we even had special names for each other. If we had such a good relationship, why was he leaving me? What had I done wrong?

After my father left, I was upset and depressed, and I began to rebel against my mother. I felt like I couldn't depend on her for the love I needed because she's not very open. She says I can talk to her, but I don't think I can. I didn't know any other way to vent my feelings, so I would keep all my anger inside and wait until she got me upset. Then I'd go off on her. I always wanted to tell her my problems and tell her what I was doing with my life, but it seemed like the older I got, the harder it was for me to tell her anything. I felt like my life was one big secret.

After my dad left, I also shrugged off all my girl friends. I felt like they couldn't do anything for me except tell me where the cute guys were going to be. They couldn't help me with my real problems. I felt like I had no one to talk to and I didn't feel close to anyone. I started to feel empty inside.

I only knew one way to fill that empty space, and that was to depend on a guy emotionally the way that I used to depend on my father. I was 12½ years old when my father left, and by my 13th birthday, I had lost my virginity. Afterwards, I wasn't proud of it, but how could I change it? It was already gone.

The first time I had sex was the biggest surprise of my life. At the time, I was mad at my boyfriend and wanted to get back at him. Another boy took me to a friend's house and we had sex in his brother's room. I had no intention of doing that. I went to our friend's house as the most naive virgin in the world, honestly thinking that nothing would happen if we were alone. Later I found out we weren't even alone: there was one guy watching from under the bed and another guy watching from the next room.

Once it was all over and the audience was gone, I didn't even know how to feel. But I didn't feel bad until I found out that the guy under the bed wanted to know if he was next.

When I got home, I went into my room and wrote in my diary. That's when it really hit me. I thought to myself, "Fetima, you just had sex with someone who doesn't even love you!" I sat there and cried. To make things worse, the guy broke up with me two days later.

I didn't have sex again for a while. I figured I wouldn't want to do it again. But when the urge did arise, I didn't fight it. I made out with all these guys who came my way, and my name was scattered all over my neighborhood.

I never really felt that I had to go all the way with them, but that's the way it happened. I had this I-don't-care attitude, but I did care even though I wouldn't admit it. I would cry every night thinking about what I was doing and how I felt. Still, I couldn't seem to change. I always wondered to myself, "What the hell is your problem? Don't you know you could catch something and die?"

I never had an answer for any of the questions that I asked myself. I felt like a lost soul walking through a graveyard, trying to find someone to take care of me, but never picking the right one. I would always go into the bedroom thinking this guy might actually like me. Then when we finished and everyone knew about it the next day, I would realize I was wrong again.

But again and again my feelings would get intertwined way too much. I'd get a big knot in my chest and think it was love. Then I would get upset with the guys when they didn't return my feelings, even though I knew deep down inside that they hardly even knew me. And the truth is that I really didn't know them either.

It's not so much that I thought that sex would lead to love, but I guess that as a girl, I thought everyone felt close after they had sex. Ten times out of 10, though, I ended up being the only one who felt something at the end of the night. I guess I just had to learn the hard way that some guys will tell you anything to keep you in their houses a little while longer.

Most people who found out what I was doing labeled me a "ho" and a "slut." They never tried to find out what was wrong, and just assumed I was doing this for the fun of it. But I never enjoyed myself. I mean, I enjoy having sex whether I like the sex or not, but mostly because I enjoy pleasing the person I'm with.

I don't know why I feel I have to satisfy other people all the time. I don't want to hurt anyone's feelings and I'm afraid they might think less of me if I don't do what they want me to do. I tend not to tell people what I truly feel. I usually just say what the person wants to hear.

For example, I was going out with a guy who made it clear he just wanted me for sex. One day I didn't feel like being bothered, but I also didn't feel like I could tell him I didn't want to have sex. So while he was in the bathroom, I just took my stuff and left. The next day I saw him driving by as I was walking home from work. He stopped the car in the middle of the street and yelled at me and called me names.

My experience with that guy made me look at my other relationships. I said to myself, "Fetima, you're so stupid!" If I'd had two other hands, I would have beat myself up.

I never knew just how badly I felt about myself until a good male friend of mine wrote me a letter telling me it was high time I took a look in the mirror and saw that I was not the person I was acting like. When I read his letter, I started to cry. I had never really thought I was a ho or a slut, because I always wanted to stay in school and make something of myself. I thought that made me different. My friend's letter made me see that I was acting like a slut, even though I knew I was worth more than that.

> **I would always go into the bedroom thinking this guy might actually like me. The next day, I would realize I was wrong again.**

The person who really helped me calm down is my current boyfriend. He and I have been together for almost three years now, even though we've argued, cheated on each other, and even broken up during that time. He has helped me realize who I am and who I want to be.

I didn't have sex with him for a whole year, as a kind of test to see if he'd wait—and he did. He wanted a serious, not just a sexual, relationship. That made me feel more confident in myself. Now I can proudly say that while I haven't made a 180 degree turnaround in my life, I have made a 90. I'm really proud of myself for that. Some people can't even make a 9 degree turn.

These days, I am still flirty and I still feel like having sex with some guys I meet (and sometimes I do). But I'm working on being monogamous. When I tell guys no, I feel proud of myself. To myself, I'm like, "You go, girl!"

I always tell younger girls that I wish I had never had sex in the first place. I know that if someone had told me that, I probably would have gone and tried it anyway. But I think it's important for girls to know that having sex with every guy, or even a select few, isn't cool. In my opinion, there is nothing wrong with having responsible sex, but if you don't want to have sex, or you don't enjoy having sex, you shouldn't do it.

When I tell guys no, I feel proud of myself.

Plus, sex is risky. Of course, you can get pregnant. And there are millions of people out there with AIDS and other diseases. We teenagers think that it's never going to happen to us. But it does!

If you're the type to call a girl names and make her feel bad—well, take it from someone who has been there, it hurts like hell. In the same time that it takes to call someone a slut or a whore, you could take some time out to talk to her. Ask her why she chooses to do the things that she does. She may be surprised at first by your asking, but I bet she will be happy that you cared enough to ask.

Fetima was 18 when she wrote this story.

Virgin Under Pressure

By Anonymous

I was excited when Jim asked me out. He'd tell me sweet things, like how he loved and cared about me and how good I looked, and how he wanted to see me every day. That made me feel like I was on top of the world.

I was also happy when Jim said that if I chose not to have sex with him, it was OK. "Finally, I met a guy who's into me but doesn't care if we have sex," I thought. It proved that he really cared about me.

I've dated about seven guys since I started high school two years ago. Not every guy I've gone out with pressured me to have sex, but it was the pushy guys I liked best because they were the ones who gave me lots of compliments and told me how much they wanted to be with me.

It's OK with me if a guy wants to have sex with me because it makes me feel desirable. But I don't like it when they really pressure me. I'm not ready to have sex yet. Most of the pushy guys I dated broke up with me when I wouldn't have sex with them. With one guy, that really hurt, because I felt attached to him.

But I'm just not ready for the consequences of sex. I'm 16 and if I got pregnant it would be a big disgrace to my family; my parents would beat me and kick me out of the house. I wouldn't want to abort if I got pregnant, but I don't want to be a teenage mother, either. I'm scared about catching an STD, too, especially since some of my friends have. I know that some STDs can cause infertility and there is no cure for HIV/AIDS.

I think the biggest thing keeping me from saying yes to sex is that I'm not ready for the emotions. I would hate to have sex with someone and then have him leave me. I'd feel used and thrown away. Also, I have guy friends who talk badly about girls they have sex with, calling them whores or sluts. I don't want to be called that, or have people see me that way. I want people to see me as someone who knows how to control herself, who respects herself, who's smart.

But another part of me does want to have sex. Part of me thinks I would really like it. Movies, TV, music, books—they make it seem like sex is heaven. I can imagine that sex would feel wonderful if I feel like the person I'm with will love me forever.

Most of my friends have already had sex, and when they talk about it, I want to experience it, too. "It feels really good," one friend told me. "If you did it once, you'd want to do it all the time." For that second, I wanted to try it. But later I reminded myself that I'm waiting for a relationship that feels more sure, and that not having sex makes me feel special because I'm not like everyone else.

But Jim, who's 20, made me feel special, too. Not a day went by when we didn't see each other or talk on the phone. I liked being with someone who made me feel good about myself.

Often I feel insecure. When I'm not dating, sometimes I feel like I'm ugly, or too fat, or just not good enough to make a guy like me. But when a guy tells me I look good, even if I think he's just sweet-talking me, I feel flattered.

Most of the time Jim and I talked on the phone because he was busy working and I had to go to school. When he wasn't busy, he came to my house. We'd just hang out for about 15 minutes before kissing and stripping. It felt good. I enjoy sexual behaviors like kissing, touching, and stripping. For me, being physical is tied up with emotions; it makes me feel more attached to the guy I'm with. I know those behaviors can lead to intercourse, but I tell myself I'll just deal with it then.

With Jim, I had about a month before I had to start dealing with it. Even though he'd told me it was OK if we didn't have sex, it started to feel like he wanted to. I noticed that he had condoms in his pocket. I started to worry about going too far.

Since I get caught up in the heat of the moment, I was afraid that one time I wouldn't say no. Also, I thought that if I said no to sex with Jim, he might get angry at me.

I wanted him to be happy with me, so he'd stay. I felt attached to him. He made me feel good about myself, and I didn't want to start over again with another guy only to have him leave me because I wouldn't have sex.

I told him, "Maybe I will have sex with you one day, but not now." I wanted Jim to think he might have a chance to have sex with me so he'd stick around.

I felt flattered that Jim wanted to have sex with me, and I liked having Jim as a boyfriend, but I still didn't feel ready.

Instead of stopping myself, or stopping Jim when things started getting really sexual, I had my friends call me when Jim was at my house. I'd discovered by accident that a ringing phone interrupts the moment and gives me a minute to think about what's going on. Then I stop whatever I'm doing and put my clothes back on.

But I wasn't sure how much longer I could keep putting off Jim—and sexual intercourse. Once, he pushed me onto the bed. At first I thought he was just playing, but he kept pushing me down.

He stopped, though, when I told him, "My mom is gonna be home very soon and you need to leave." I was relieved; his forcefulness had surprised me. I was angry with Jim for pushing me down on the bed like that. But the next day, he called me at 8 a.m. and asked me how I was feeling. It made me think he still cared about me, and that reassured me.

I told myself that he should know that I wasn't ready to have sex with him. But when I look back at it now, I realize that I didn't say anything to him directly about not wanting to have sex—I always made excuses, like my mom was going to come home, or that maybe I'd be ready one day, or I had my friends call me.

He didn't try to force me to do anything after that, but all we talked about on the phone was sex. He'd tell me how he couldn't wait to have sex with me and how he wanted to be my first. If it made him happy to talk about sex, instead of actually having sex, that was fine with me. We could talk about sex all he wanted—I just didn't want to do it.

But when he said things like, "We're gonna have sex the next time I come to your house," I felt like I didn't want him to come over. I was afraid that he might actually try it, and I didn't want to be in that situation. I felt flattered that Jim wanted to have sex with me, and I liked having Jim as a boyfriend, but I still didn't feel ready.

Over the summer, the pressure got more intense, to the point that I got scared to go to his house or for him to come to mine. Finally I told him outright, "I'm not ready to have sex," but he said that if I had sex with him I wouldn't regret it because it would be the best sex I would ever have.

I was confused. I remembered how he'd told me that it was OK if I didn't have sex with him and wondered what had changed. I felt that he was the one changing—but was he becoming the real him? I felt like I wouldn't have gone out with him if he was going to give me that much pressure. But I couldn't bring myself to break up with him, either. I still liked the attention and thought I'd get lonely without him.

In August, he called and asked me to come over. Even though I felt unsure, I went because I wanted to please him. As soon as I walked in the living room, he started kissing me and taking off my clothes. Soon we were on his bed kissing, and he was touching me everywhere, which I enjoyed. Then I felt something trying to push in me, and he said, "Don't worry, I have a condom on."

I felt helpless and surprised. "Don't worry?" I thought. "Did I tell you that I wanted to have sex with you? If I wanted to have sex, it sure as hell wouldn't be with you." At that minute, I had no desire to have sex with him. I hated him. I told him, "Please get off me, please."

Then he asked me, "Are you scared?"

"Yes."

"Don't worry. If you want me to stop in the middle of it, I will." But as he was talking, he was trying to push his penis in me. I was trying to close my legs.

I thought, "Oh God, please let me leave this house still a virgin, and if I get back to my house I will never step foot in this house again."

I begged him to get off me. He was angry, but he did. I was so relieved. I just wanted to leave. But I also felt bad for not having sex with him, because he'd waited longer than most guys I dated and I wanted to make him happy and make him stay with me.

So when he asked me if I wanted to sleep next to him on the bed, I said yes. Even though he'd made me mad, I wanted to please him because I'd upset him by pushing him away. I put on my underwear and lay next to him, imagining he respected my decision not to have sex. I wanted to believe that I could trust him.

He started touching me again, which I didn't care about as long as he didn't try to have sex. But he did. As I tried to shove him off, he kept trying to force himself on me. Then I shoved harder.

This didn't feel like the sex that goes with love; I felt like he was trying to rape me. I was angry. I thought I'd made it clear that I didn't want to have sex, and he was still trying to do it. I shoved back, and seconds later he got up, angry again. This time I didn't care anymore if he was angry or not because I just wanted to leave. So I got up, put on my clothes and left him sitting on the bed.

I still felt like I loved him, but I also felt very angry at him. I wondered if he'd break up with me since I didn't have sex with him. But he kept calling me, and we both pretended that nothing had happened. I didn't bring it up because I didn't want to get him angry again. The conversations felt normal, and I was happy about that; he ended the calls telling me he loved me, and I told him, "I love you too." Two days later, I even let him come to my house, and we fooled around like we usually did. I felt good that things were back on track. But I trusted him less.

Over the next few weeks, I saw less of him. I began to suspect that I wasn't the only girl he was seeing. He wouldn't pick up the phone when I called him, and when I did talk to him, he gave me excuses about being busy. That made me doubt that he still loved me. I felt stupid, and I decided to break up with him.

A couple of weeks later I saw him standing outside with his friends. I told him that I didn't want to go out with him any longer. He asked me why, and I said that I just didn't. If I gave him a reason he would have tried to please me and give me excuses. I didn't want any reasons; I just wanted to leave him.

I wasn't used to breaking up with guys. Usually they were the ones who broke up with me. But I felt proud of myself because I finally had the guts to end a relationship I wasn't happy with. I am still not sure about sex, but if I'm going to have sex with someone, I'd have to trust him more as time goes on, not less.

I want to be confident enough to tell a guy clearly that I'm not ready to have sex without being so afraid that he'll leave me.

I feel lonely without a boyfriend, especially when I have no one to call at night, but I don't want to go out for a while. My experience with Jim made me wonder why I wanted to please guys so badly, and why I didn't think about myself more.

I've started thinking, "What about me? What's wrong with me that I keep thinking about pleasing him? What about pleasing myself?" It made sense to me at the time, but now I don't know why pleasing a guy was so important to me.

So now I'm trying to figure out what I want. I'd like a long relationship. I don't want to see a boyfriend just once in a while. I want to spend a lot of time with him and do things together. I'd like to be with someone who's confident. We can argue about things—that's OK, even fun sometimes, as long as no one gets really mad and curses. But I also want him to respect me and listen when I say I don't want to do something. And I want to be confident enough to tell a guy clearly that I'm not ready to have sex without being so afraid that he'll leave me.

What's best for me right now is to learn to be independent, and not care that my friends have boyfriends, or feel lonely because I don't have one. I want to stop comparing myself to others. It only makes me feel inadequate, and that makes me vulnerable to guys when they flatter me.

I hope that when summer comes around again, I'll have learned my lesson and will feel happy being independent. I don't want another summer of pressure.

The author was in high school when she wrote this story.
After graduation she enrolled in college.

I Wasn't Pressured

By Anonymous

Most girls seem to think that guys are only out for one thing. In my experience, that's not true. Not all guys are out there to "hit it and split."

Like my boyfriend, John. He is nice, sweet, and he seems to care about what's on my mind. In the beginning of our relationship, he always told me, "Sex ain't got nothing to do with it, 'cause I ain't going nowhere." I believed him, and when we did start having sex, it was because I wanted to.

I met John (not his real name) in the 8th grade and we began dating at the end of June. I was expecting our relationship to last about a month. My best friend was just starting to date a boy also and she and I were making bets on how long both of our relationships would last. We gave both our relationships till August 31. We were getting ready to enter high school and thinking you can't be tied down with a boyfriend when you're starting a new school.

But somehow, my relationship with John lasted the whole summer. I did have suspicions that he was going to break up with me in the fall because we were going to different schools, but we overcame that. After I saw that our relation-

Not all guys are out there to "hit it and split."

ship was going to last, I started planning to have sex with John. I thought about doing it when I turned 16, because that seemed like the right age, or maybe on our one-year anniversary. I felt John was the right one because our relationship lasted so long. Before him, I had only dated guys for a week or two, and we never even talked about having sex.

J ohn and I did talk about it, but he wasn't begging me to have sex. He never pressured me to do anything, even though I know he really wanted it. His friends were the ones asking me, "When you gonna let him blaze?" They made me feel bad about it.

When John and I would hear songs with sexual lyrics, we would look at each other and laugh, or he would try to be funny and say, "We don't have to listen to that." About seven months into our relationship, I felt it was time to have sex with John. I didn't think I could wait until our anniversary. It was just something I felt like doing. I always thought about it, so I decided to act upon it.

The first time we had sex was in his room. The only thing going through my mind was if it was going to hurt. He tried to relax me by doing some freaky things. He seemed to know what he was doing, which made me wonder how many other times he had done this. He told me he had done it twice before but with the same girl and that she was 17.

John and I are still together and our relationship has been going nicely so far. Sex has become an important part of our relationship and we try to be safe about it by always using protection.

Having sex has made us closer. Now we talk to each other better and we understand each other more. We seem to play around with each other more. We say whatever comes out of our mouths about each other and I feel more comfortable around him than I did in the beginning of our relationship.

People may read this and say that I'm too young and I don't know any better and I should have waited. But I feel that having sex with John was the right thing to do. I don't regret it because this was something I wanted.

The author was in high school when she wrote this story.

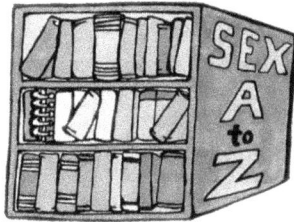

Chapter 2

Six Things to Ask About 'Doing It'

Have you masturbated?

Some people don't feel the need to masturbate, don't feel comfortable with it, or just don't enjoy it. But many, many others—male and female, gay and straight, whether virgins or sexually active, single or in a relationship—do it and like it.

If you're not sure you're ready to get sexual with another person, masturbating is a great alternative. It will help you figure out how and where you like to be touched, what gets you excited and what doesn't. It will relieve feelings of sexual tension and horniness without putting you at risk for sexually transmitted

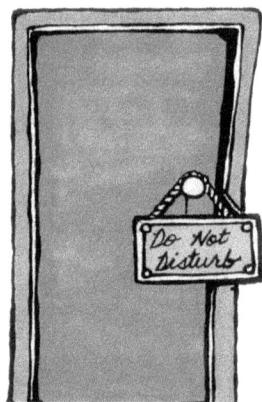

diseases, pregnancy, or a broken heart. Best of all, it feels good.

You may have heard that masturbation is "unnatural," "sick," or just plain "gross." Nothing could be further from the truth. Masturbating is totally normal. Or you may have heard that masturbating will make you go blind, grow hair on your palms, break out, become sterile, or go insane. None of this is true either

So relax. Masturbating won't hurt you. What it will do is make you more knowledgeable about and comfortable with your body and your sexuality.

Do you know the facts about sex? Do you know what to do?

While it's true that sex comes naturally (if people *had* to read a book to figure it out, none of us would be here today), it's also true that you can learn things about sex without actually having it. How do you learn? For one thing, you can read books or search online for information that tells you the basic facts about sex and your body. (See p. 311 for some helpful books and websites.) That way you can sort out what's false and what's true.

But there are other ways to learn, too. You can fantasize about doing it (which can help you figure out what gets you excited). You can practice on yourself. You can talk to people you trust: your best friend or favorite cousin, your parents (if you think they can handle it), your partner.

You can also read erotic novels or websites, or talk to friends who have had sex already about what the actual experience is like. While there's something to be learned from all of these sources, keep in mind that when it comes to personal stories about sex, people tend to exaggerate and even out-and-out lie about what they've done, how often they've done it, who they've done it with, and how it felt. The "true life" stories that appear online or in magazines like *Cosmo*, and even the stories your friends tell you, are often full of what people *wish* had happened, rather than the reality of their experiences. And porn, in particular, is exaggerated and fake. No matter what the site or magazine may claim, you're watching actors performing (or being exploited), not real-life people having consensual sex. So don't let what you see, read, or hear make you feel inadequate or insecure.

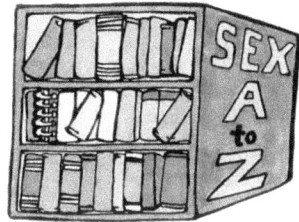

Seek information from the most trustworthy sources you can find, but remember—in the end, the only thing that counts is that you and your partner enjoy being together and are caring and responsible. It'll help if you talk to each other about your experiences with sex so far; what you've liked and haven't liked, what you want (or don't want) to try.

Do you know what kind of contraception you and your partner might use and how to get it?

If you're not actively trying to have a baby, you need to be actively trying *not* to get pregnant. There are lots of ways to do that. Be aware, however, that only condoms (when used correctly) protect you from sexually transmitted diseases. Always use a condom for disease protection, in addition to other forms of birth control to prevent pregnancy.

In order to *use* contraception, you have to get it, and know how to use it properly. This involves a little planning. (For more information on the different kinds of birth control methods, see p. 280.)

Before you can use a condom, for example, you have to have one handy (which means you have to walk into a store and buy some or ask for them at school or at a local clinic). You also have to know how to put it on. (For more on buying and using condoms, see p. 281.)

It's a good idea to visit your doctor or a sexual health clinic, like Planned Parenthood, before you have sex. A doctor or nurse practitioner can talk with you about your options for birth control, answer any questions you have, make sure you're healthy, and give you condoms and any birth control prescriptions you need.

Don't wait until you're about to do it to ask, "Do you have something?" or "Are you using anything?"

Would you know if you had an STD? Are you prepared to get tested regularly?

Unfortunately, sex can be hazardous to your health. Sexually Transmitted Diseases (STDs—also called Sexually Transmitted Infections, or STIs) can range from annoying and embarrassing (pubic lice) to potentially life-threatening (HIV and syphilis). Symptoms can take a long time to develop or be barely noticeable; some people can be infected and not develop symptoms.

The best way to protect yourself from STDs is to use a condom and/or dental dam whenever you have sex. (Dental dams are pieces of latex that are used to form a barrier between the mouth and vagina or anus during oral sex.) The more people you or your partner have sex with, the greater the risk of catching an STD—especially if you don't use protection every time.

If you're sexually active, be vigilant about checking yourself and your partner for possible STD symptoms (and you need to do this when the lights are on!). Symptoms include lumps, bumps, or sores in the genital area, burning during urination, unusual vaginal discharge, and inflammation or swelling of the scrotum (balls). If you have any of these symptoms, visit your doctor or a free public health clinic and get checked out. And don't have sex again until you get the results.

But since some STDs are hard or even impossible to detect, the only way to be absolutely sure you don't have one is to be tested regularly. Doctors generally recommend that sexually active teens get tested twice a year—more often if you have several different partners (or are sleeping with someone who has, or had, a lot of different partners). Sometimes teens are so frightened by the thought that they might have an STD that they never get tested. But that puts themselves and their partners at risk.

If you do get tested and have an STD, you need to tell your partner(s) so they can be checked as well. Telling someone they may have an STD can be a hard thing to do. But most STDs can be cured with medication and even those that can't be cured can be treated. Many people with HIV, for example, are living longer, healthier lives today than they did 20 years ago because of the new drugs that have become available. (See p. 293 for more about STDs.) No matter how hard it is to tell, if you don't tell you're risking your partner's health and increasing the chance that they'll spread disease. You'd want someone to tell you, right?

What if you had sex without protection, or the condom breaks? What would you do next?

You might want to panic, cry, or pretend it didn't happen. But if you don't want to get pregnant, there's something more constructive you can do. It's called Emergency Contraception (EC)—also known as the "morning after pill" or Plan B. EC reduces your chances of getting pregnant if you take it within 120 hours (five days) of having unprotected sex, although it's most effective if you take it within 72 hours (three days). You can get it from your gynecologist, local hospital, or Planned Parenthood clinic (some cities also offer EC at STD clinics). But you have to act fast. The sooner you take EC, the better it works to prevent a pregnancy.

If you don't know of any doctors or clinics you can go to, call 1-888-NOT-2-LATE for a list of emergency contraception providers near you. You can call at any hour of the day

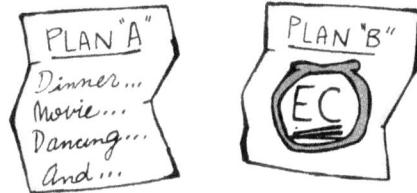

PLAN "A"
Dinner...
Movie....
Dancing...
And...

PLAN "B"
EC

or night. Based on the phone number you're calling from, a recorded announcement will give you the names and phone numbers of five places where you can get EC in your area. Then you have to call the providers, say you want emergency contraception, and make an appointment. (For more information on EC and how it works, see p. 291.)

EC won't protect you from contracting HIV or any other STD. If you've had unprotected sex or were using a condom and it broke, make sure that you and your partner both get tested for STDs, including an HIV test. Many public health clinics offer free and confidential testing.

Have you looked at pornography? How has it affected the way you view sex?

Pornography is so easily available on the Internet that you almost cannot avoid it. Nowadays it's likely that you and/or your partner will have some experience with pornography.

But what does pornography have to do with sex? Some pornography is erotic. It's shows people stimulating each other in loving and caring ways. There's probably nothing wrong with that, and if you're inexperienced with sex you might even learn something from it.

But most pornography has little to do with sex. Instead, it is designed to appeal to people who get off on violence, or on seeing other people (especially women) get degraded. Treating people violently, or degrading them, is inappropriate in any relationship, including a sexual one.

Another problem with pornography is that it is fake. It is performed by actors with unusual or surgically altered bodies, who are often also taking drugs to help them perform. One of the worst effects of pornography is that some people think it's real and feel inadequate because they don't look or perform like porn stars.

Finally, lots of porn shows unsafe sex. Porn actors are often desperate young people—youth who've been abused and are homeless or runaways. The porn industry, which is hugely profitable, exploits these actors, and often forces them to perform unsafe acts. Sexually transmitted diseases, including HIV, are common in the industry.

If your partner wants you to do something because he "saw it in a porn movie," that's a warning sign that it could be violent, degrading, unsafe, or impossible.

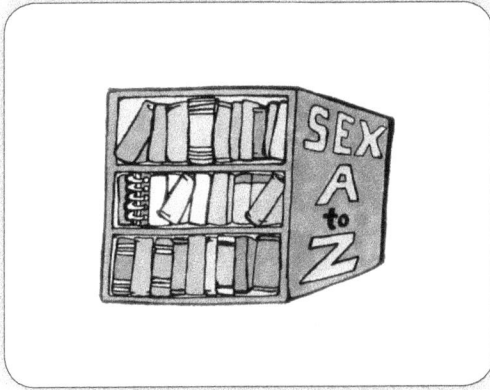

Learning About Sex

Teens Share Their Experiences

Infatuation With Masturbation

Why is enjoying our bodies so shameful?

By Tasha

I didn't know what an orgasm was until I was 12. The word "cum" came up in a music video and I wondered, "What's that? Why don't I have one?"

I asked my sister what "cum" meant and she said, "It means orgasm."

"What's an orgasm?"

"I don't know. I can't describe it. It's when you're having sex and then you cum."

"Oh," I said, trying to sound sophisticated. Really, I had no idea what the hell she was talking about. I looked it up in the dictionary: "**Orgasm:** noun. the highest point of sexual tension." That told me nothing except that I would have to have sex to experience this orgasm and I wasn't having sex anytime soon. I wondered if there was another way to have one.

A year later, I was in the library walking around when I found a book called *Deal With It*, about girls' sexuality, minds, and bodies. I was drawn in by the cover, which had a picture of a girl wearing an open raincoat over a bikini.

I soon got to a two-page spread, literally—a drawing of a girl opening her legs to reveal all of her girlness. The in-depth diagram pointed out the clitoris, the vulva and the pubic hair, among other things. Wow! When I got to the part about the clitoris—the nerve center of girls' sexual pleasure, and something I never knew I had—I was transfixed with the idea of exploring it.

It took two days for me to muster up the courage to try. I was afraid that it would hurt, or that my mom would come in and think I was being disgusting.

But one day I lay down on my bed and decided I would do it. First I touched my breasts to warm up. Soon I felt comfortable and began playing with my clitoris. I loved it! I finally got my orgasm. My infatuation with masturbation began.

After that I kept...exploring. Sometimes even three times a day! Blush. I was always worried that my mother or one of my sisters would walk in on me mid-passion and think I was being disgusting. (They have—they gave me funny looks and acted like they didn't see anything. They should learn to knock.) They're deeply religious and think that sexuality is disgusting outside of marriage.

I began wondering why masturbation is something everyone does but no one will admit to, like farting in a crowded room.

Once in 9th grade, I was sitting in the cafeteria with my girlfriends when the subjects of sex and masturbation came up. One friend asked me if I had ever masturbated. I said, "Yeah, a lot." But when I asked her, she just turned deaf and ignored me.

I thought that was weird because we were being so open just moments before. Besides, masturbating is healthy and normal. Why is enjoying your body so uncomfortable and embarrassing in our society?

By last year, I was fed up with the taboo that tells us to do it in the darkest corners and, if ever asked, deny, deny, deny. To investigate why it exists, I handed out a survey in my school, Edward R. Murrow HS, to about 150 people ages 14-21. It surprised me how quickly word got around about what I was doing.

Most people delightedly took the survey, some said no and others just gave me b.s. answers. It was anonymous, which I think helped most people speak openly. I couldn't wait to get back to the office and read the responses with my editor. The answers confirmed what I'd suspected— masturbation is fine to do, but not to discuss.

Most people said they masturbated and enjoyed it. One girl said that afterwards she felt "relieved, exhausted, and ready to focus on my daily life." A boy said, "I feel relaxed and happy. Sometimes I even cry because I am so happy." I couldn't tell if he was bs-ing or not, but he wrote a lot so I'm taking him at his word.

But despite their enjoyment, most people I surveyed said they were embarrassed by masturbation and said it's not an open topic in their homes or among friends. A surprising few did say they're open about it, including some who said, "Hell, yeah!" One guy wrote, "Yes, of course, every member of my family masturbates on occasion." But they were the exceptions.

I began wondering why masturbation is something everyone does but no one will admit to, like farting in a crowded room.

Most teens said they learned about masturbation through word of mouth, on their own, by watching porn, reading books, or talking to friends. No one said they heard about it on TV, in sex education class or by communicating with adults (except one boy, but that's one out of 150).

Maybe that's why there are so many euphemisms for masturbation, like "jerkin' off," "spankin' the monkey" and "petting the bunny." Using cutesy words is a good way to disguise your discomfort with a subject.

But the survey didn't answer my biggest question: why do teens talk about sex openly—and adults talk to us about sex, at least in sex ed—but masturbation is completely off limits?

Maybe it's because some religious people say masturbation is wrong, or because some people see it as something only desperate people in need of sex do. Maybe it's because most of our movie heroes and music stars only portray healthy sexuality as getting it on with other people.

It seems to me that many people think that exploring your sexuality is OK as long as someone else is doing the exploring. Society is saying, "It's OK to touch other people but not yourself."

That's funny, because society also tells us, "Love yourself or no one else will." How about putting those words into practice and loving yourself physically, too?

To me, masturbation is part of finding out more about my sexuality. I want to find out what I like sexually by exploring myself. When I fool around with someone, I want to be able to feel comfortable saying what I like and don't like. I like being able to tell my partner exactly where and how I want to be touched.

I also like having control over my body and my pleasure, knowing that I don't need to get caught up in someone else to feel good. To me, masturbation isn't an alternative to sex. It's something enjoyable and fun that I can do for myself.

The author was 17 when she wrote this story. She later graduated high school, served as an Americorps volunteer, and went to college, studying sociology.

Learning Without Doing
How I Kept My Head About Sex

By Nadishia Forbes

When I was a little kid—6, 7, probably even 8 years old—sex was a mystery. I was a child with a big imagination and I used to think that a girl could get pregnant after kissing a boy.

Later, when I was 9, 10 and 11, I was enlightened by my friends, who told me sex was allowing a boy to stick his penis into your vagina. Of course, with this information came the school rumors of little boys and girls having sex in the bushes, in the classroom, behind the building, and wherever else they could think of.

Even though we thought sex was nasty and were embarrassed by it, we also found it mysterious and interesting. We assumed it was one of the things adults did for fun, like kissing and drinking beer, but we wanted to know more. I wasn't getting any sex education in school. And the only grown-up person who used to talk to me about sex was my grandmother's stepdaughter. She would tell my cousin and me not to have sex and she would give us a little information about menstruation, but not enough to be much help.

When I was 13, I moved in with my grandmother. During my first two years with her, she talked to me about boys and sex no more than two or three times. What she had to say was either confusing or negative, so I didn't gain much from our discussions. What she was clear about was that I couldn't go to parties, date, or have boyfriends. She explained that if I did those things, something could happen to me that I might later regret.

My grandmother needn't have worried about me. I definitely wasn't interested in having sex at that point. Most of the older women in my life, including my grandmother, had gotten pregnant while they were in their teens. That fact, along with my grandmother's lectures, made me feel that if I had any type of relationship—even a friendship—with a boy, I would eventually get pregnant or become a slut. Besides that, I am a Christian and was raised to believe that having sex outside of marriage is sinful and dirty.

Probably because of my grandmother's influence, I started my teens feeling nervous and uncomfortable around boys. But, like any teenager, I was also curious and wanting to know about sex. My body was changing and I was having a lot of crushes, even though I didn't act on them. I had a lot of questions. Nobody had even told me exactly what my period was.

At the library one day when I was 14, I saw a book that had the word "period" written on it. I was eager to learn more about menstruation, so I read it. It helped me to understand what my body was going through.

The more I read, the more I wanted to know. I read about periods, puberty, and sex. One time I saw a book with a bunch of naked people of all sizes in it. I couldn't believe they had a book like that in the children's section of the library. The book talked about having sex, what the man does and what the woman does. It even had a picture of a naked couple under the sheets. I was surprised and a little shocked, but curiosity and excitement took over. As I read, I felt like a bandit stealing secrets.

From books, I learned a lot of the facts about sex, pregnancy, and STDs.

From books, I learned a lot of the facts about sex, pregnancy, and STDs, but I still had questions about what the actual experience was like. I would ask my uncle's 18-year-old girlfriend and my 15-year-old friend about what it was like when they lost their virginity. "Did it hurt?" and "At what age did you lose it?" were my main questions. One girl told me that having sex felt like menstrual cramps; another told me it hurt at first but felt better later.

None of this information made me eager to try it myself, so all through junior high, I continued avoiding all boys. I was very shy and nervous talking to them. I didn't want to be seen with guys, especially at church, where people might think that my wild, teenage hormones were on the loose and conclude that I was having sex.

Then, when I started high school, I decided it was time to get myself a boyfriend. Sex wasn't in my plans. The idea of having sex was still quite scary. But everyone else seemed to have a boyfriend and they would show off about it, so I wanted one too. I wanted to know what it was like to be in a relationship.

One day when I was going to class I noticed this boy kept looking at me. Thinking he was cute and this could be my chance to get a boyfriend, I called him over. This was really brave for someone as shy as I was, but my determination enabled me to overcome my anxiety. We started going out that day.

We didn't have much in common and, besides his looks, there wasn't anything I liked about him. Going out with someone I didn't like was a mistake. When we kissed for the first time, it felt disgusting. I wasn't attracted to him at all, which is why it was easy to say no when he asked me to have sex with him. My curiosity was replaced with fear and disgust. We had only been going out for two weeks when he tried to talk me into it. I got mad and went home and didn't speak to him again.

I met someone I was attracted to about a year later, when I was almost 16. He was in my Spanish class and I started hanging out with him. One day, we went down into his basement and talked. After a while, he asked for a kiss. I was nervous but I wrapped my arms around his neck and kissed him. Then he drew me closer to him. It was all very exciting, but then he went into the corner of the basement and said, "Come here." I got scared, quickly made up an excuse, and left. We kissed one time after that but I decided I definitely couldn't handle even the thought of sex, let alone sex itself.

After that, I lost interest in boys for a while. I was quite busy maturing and learning. Then I met this guy named Dave at church. He was a tall, broad-shouldered, good-looking guy. A lot of times, I would see him looking at me, and eventually I gave him my phone number.

Some time later he called and I had fun talking to him. I told him I liked him and he told me how good I looked in my tight skirt. He also kept insisting on coming over to my house and asking me if I had my own room. I started getting suspicious and thinking, "The only reason why a guy would be so eager to get to my room is if he was hoping to have sex."

At the time he started calling me, I was a little depressed and I had problems both at school and with my parents. But when I tried to tell Dave about my problems, he wasn't any help at all. I was looking for someone to talk to, someone who would care about me and understand me. All he seemed to want was sex.

I think that going out and getting a lot of information about sex during my early teens has helped me to postpone doing it.

I'm 18 now and I still haven't had sex. And I still don't feel ready. I think that going out and getting a lot of information about sex during my early teens has helped me to postpone doing it. I got to understand that sex can be a wonderful or a dangerous experience.

My grandmother tried to influence me by only telling me about the dangerous part and maybe that made me more frightened of boys than I needed to be. I wish she could have just been straight with me and said, "Even though I don't want you to have sex because of its dangers, it's your decision. If you choose not to have sex, it will be a little hard to resist sometimes because you're maturing into a woman and you're gonna have feelings that you may not understand. Just be careful and you can come to me whenever you have questions."

It's lucky that I'm one of those people who actually enjoys reading. I was able to learn a lot about sex from books. If I hadn't known the facts, I probably would have had sex already because of my curiosity, without knowing the risks. But with knowledge comes the wisdom to make good choices.

Nadishia was a senior in high school when she wrote this story. She graduated and joined the Army, where she became a Biological Warfare Specialist. She later had a daughter.

How to Buy a Condom

By Cassaundra Worrell

The big day came. I was going to buy some condoms—and the only way I felt comfortable about it was to buy them in a different neighborhood. I walked into a large pharmacy where I figured I could remain anonymous. I laughed to myself, certain that no one had spotted me. Little did I know.

Beads of sweat formed across my brow. I waited as the area around the cash register slowly emptied before I approached. In a timid voice I asked for the intimidating item. A slow grin spread across the cashier's face. He then asked in a booming voice, "Lubricated or dry?"

When I said "Yes," he realized he had yet another victim. He went for the kill. By now I was ready to crack, because there was a line of people waiting behind me. With that menacing grin, he screamed, "Ribbed or regular, colored or clear, flavored or without taste, lambskin or latex, edible or non-edible, and what size box?"

By this time I was ready to make in my pants. "Regular, please, and the largest box you have." I added the last part so I would never have to come back.

I got the courage to look him in the face and saw that his name tag said "Mike." Mike's face got red from laughter as he told me the condoms were kept in aisle four.

Am I the only one who has gone through the trauma of purchasing condoms? My classmates who will read this may wonder how I managed. "Weren't you afraid that someone would laugh at you?" It was degrading to have "Mike" laugh in my face and to have the people on line behind me look at me with "shame, shame, shame" written across their foreheads. But I survived, and you can, too.

I know that buying a condom can be rough the first time, but at least you are taking responsibility for your actions, and it could just save your life. Think about this as you ask for that box of condoms—being embarrassed is much better than being dead.

Cassaundra was in high school when she wrote this story.
She later graduated from college and became a nurse.

My Best Friend Has an STD

By Anonymous

There's not a day when I don't talk to my friend Shalane. We talk about school, our family problems, boyfriend issues. Even though she's had sex and I don't want to yet, we understand each other.

We used to talk about people who have STDs and how stupid they were for not protecting themselves. I didn't think I knew anyone with an STD. Then, one night last summer, Shalane called me. She was in the hospital.

"Hey, what's wrong with you?" I said.

"I am not feeling well, obviously," she snapped.

"Don't try to play smart with me. What happened?"

"I have PID," she said. "It felt like I had cramps. But they were hurting so bad, my mother took me to the emergency room."

"So what is PID?" I asked.

Shalane explained to me that PID is pelvic inflammatory disease. It affects a woman's reproductive organs, mainly the uterus. She told me she had chlamydia, an STD. Because she didn't know she had it—often chlamydia doesn't have symptoms—she didn't get treatment, and it spread, causing the PID. As a result, even though she was only 16, she might not be able to have kids anymore.

At first I thought she was just fooling around, because we sometimes play around with things like that. But she was serious. I felt shocked because to me STDs didn't exist.

I knew that sometimes Shalane didn't use condoms because she'd told me. But as far as I knew she only took that chance with one guy, Trey. Still, I knew she'd had three or four boyfriends she'd had sex with. So I asked her who she thought she got it from. She said she didn't know.

In my mind I was thinking, "I wish you were more like me when it comes to sex. Then you wouldn't be going through this. I don't have sex because I think I can't handle the consequences."

But I didn't say that to Shalane because I didn't want to hurt her feelings. She was already feeling bad. Instead, I changed the topic. Truthfully, I didn't feel comfortable talking about it. I didn't want her feeling like I was judging her because of her disease.

Besides, I understood how she could have done it. Even though I tell myself I'd be sure to use a condom if I had sex, I can see myself doing the same thing as Shalane if I got caught up in the heat of the moment. That's why I think it's safer for me to tell my boyfriend that I won't have sex with him—even though that's not easy either.

The next morning, Shalane called me, crying. Just hearing her cry made me sadder than I was before. I asked her what was wrong, and she asked me to call Trey. She thought he might have been the one that gave her chlamydia. Trey was the first boyfriend she had sex with. Even though they'd broken up, they were still friends—and sometimes still had sex. I agreed to call Trey, but he wasn't home. When I told Shalane she started crying more. I felt terrible, and rushed to the hospital to see her.

When I got to her room she was watching TV, ready to eat her breakfast. I was happy to see her with a smile on her face, because when she called me she sounded like she was dying. I sat on her hospital bed and we started talking.

She told me that she was angry at herself for maybe not being able to have kids. She wasn't planning on having one any time soon, but she had often told me that she wanted to have a child someday. I felt bad for her and I was kind of angry at myself, too, that I hadn't tried harder to convince her not to have sex.

A few weeks later, Shalane asked Trey if he had an STD, but he said he went to the doctor recently and everything was fine. Shalane believed him. They're friends and she didn't think there was any reason for him to lie. But if it wasn't Trey who gave it to her, who was it? All of her exes looked fine. As it turns out, chlamydia—the most common sexually transmitted infection in the U.S.—often has no symptoms in males, either.

Shalane decided not to ask the other guys she had had sex with. She thought that they'd say no, even though that would mean one of them was lying. But what really stopped her from asking was that if she did, they would know that she had an STD, and then they might tell other people. She trusted Trey to keep a secret, but she couldn't trust the others.

I didn't think I knew anyone with an STD. Then Shalane called me from the hospital.

She worried that people would start view-ing her as a whore, because around where I live, that's how people talk about females with STDs. It's not fair, but there are names for girls who have an STD but no name for a guy who has an STD.

I think she cares more about her reputation than about who gave it to her or who they might give it to. Finding the person who gave it to her won't cure the disease—antibiotics killed it—and it won't change her ability to have children.

If she talked to her other ex-boyfriends about her chlamydia, they might find that they have it too, and get it cured before it turns into something worse or before they spread it to someone else. But she's not going to. I know it's cold to say that you don't care about other people, but I think I'd do the same thing to protect myself from possible shame and social humiliation.

Of course, that's how STDs are spread. Someone who doesn't know he has an STD has sex without a condom and gives it to his partner. Or someone knows or suspects he has an STD, but he just wants to have sex and doesn't care to tell his partner that he's infected.

Honest communication could go a long way toward slowing the

spread of STDs. But it's a hard thing to talk about. In my relationships, I haven't started up a conversation about STDs because I just don't feel comfortable talking about them. I'm also afraid my boyfriend will think I don't trust him.

The problem is that no one really wants to talk about STDs or think about them. I didn't talk about it seriously with Shalane or my friends before she got PID. I didn't think we would ever be affected.

The author was in high school when she wrote this story.

The Morning After

By Anonymous

I'm a 20-year-old black female from New York attending a university in the South. I first started having sex during my freshman year and have continued to be sexually active. I liked having casual sex, partly because I found on-campus relationships too complicated.

I'd recently met a guy, Dante, who I liked. Dante had decent looks and a good sense of humor. He was in the Army, majoring in civil engineering at a historically black college nearby. He took pride in being a black man doing big things, and that's very sexy to me.

I'd been seeing Dante for a couple of weeks when I called him over to my apartment on a Friday night during booty-call hours (any time between midnight and dawn). I supplied the liquor and he hooked up the movies. I had a few drinks because I was feeling so antsy. I was soon buzzed.

We finished one movie and then started to watch another. It felt like we were waiting to devour each other. We never finished watching the second movie. I was prepared, and had the condoms by the bedpost.

Only, that night, Dante had a hard time keeping his erection. We tried putting on the condom, but he shrank again. That's when I made a decision that I later came to regret: I decided to start having intercourse with him without a condom. I figured we could put on the condom after he was able to stay erect.

Granted, this is risky behavior—as I soon found out, it can be hard to stop sex once you get started. And not using a condom means possibly exposing yourself to STDs. But that night, I decided to take a chance. Dante maintained his arousal and then entered me. At this point, I thought to stop him and put on a condom, but I didn't. I was buzzed, and also didn't want to break the rhythm we'd finally achieved. The night was finally taking off. I was caught up in the moment.

That is, until he strained out an anguished shout that came just after he did. We'd only been having sex for a few minutes. With a look of pleasure mixed with fright, he lay down beside me.

"I just came," he said, breathing heavily. "Are you on birth control?"

"No," I said.

There was silence. I was determined not to panic. I wanted to wait until I was a little more sober and could sort everything out. So I went to sleep and let him spend the night. With hugs and a kiss, we parted later that morning with an, "I'll be in touch." He sheepishly nodded and left. I knew I wasn't going to call him again.

I played the night's events back over in my mind. In my head were the excuses I'd heard from other girls who didn't think their risky behavior could get them pregnant: "It happened too quickly." "He wasn't in long at all."

I remembered sitting through the health lectures in high school and freshman year of college and the TV specials, thinking, "At this point, who doesn't know that unprotected sex can equal pregnancy or worse?" And here I was trying to convince myself that I couldn't be pregnant even though I'd just had unsafe sex!

I had homework to do, errands to run, and friends to catch up with, so I convinced myself not to worry. But I was two, maybe three weeks into my menstrual cycle, which is the time when women are most likely to get pregnant. Thoughts of my stupid actions and possible pregnancy seeped into my head in my apartment, at the food-court, in the library, and in between friends' conversations.

I couldn't take a chance and wait to see if I was pregnant. I knew what I had to do. I would take the morning after pill—more appropriately called the up-to-five-days-after pill. One of my high school friends had a pregnancy scare a year ago and did a lot of research on emergency contraception, as it's called.

She told me how it worked. I had 72 hours (three days) to take the pill and have a good chance of it working. (You can take emergency contraception up to five days after having sex, but the sooner you take it, the more effective it is). The pill tricks your reproductive system into believing you're already pregnant. The body then builds a defense system to block a fertilized egg from setting in your uterus.

Unfortunately, it was Saturday and the school's health clinic wasn't open until Monday. I worried about waiting two days. The more I tried to push negative thoughts out of my mind, the more they pushed back.

I didn't want to wait things out and see if I turned up pregnant. I'd always assumed that if I had an unwanted pregnancy, I would have an abortion. But now that the possibility seemed real, I worried that abortion would feel like murder. At the same time, I had no desire to be anyone's mother. Having a child would wreck my chances of achieving my goals.

My worry was like a little snowball that got bigger and bigger as it rolled down the hills of my mind. I regretted having unprotected sex and being at the mercy of the weekend. I spent the rest of the weekend doing homework, waiting. I just wanted to get to Monday, get my pill, and move on.

At 8:30 Monday morning, I made an appointment over the phone with the student clinic to get the morning after pill. A million thoughts passed through my mind in the hour between the call and my appointment.

"Should I tell Dante what I'm doing?" I wondered. "And could I tell my mom?"

"No," I told myself. If I took the pill, I wouldn't get pregnant. I wouldn't tell Dante because we hadn't been a couple and didn't have a major emotional attachment. He hadn't even called to see if I was OK.

As for Mom, I wanted her to think that I'm safe. From this point on, I knew I would be, and didn't see any reason to upset her. It would be hard for me to forgive myself for disappointing her over something as seemingly simple as safer sex.

At the clinic, a nurse saw me first. While taking my blood pressure and body temperature, she asked me if the sex was consensual, if I'd failed to use a condom or if it had broken, and if I was on birth control. A few minutes later, Dr. M. entered.

I couldn't take a chance and wait to see if I was pregnant. I knew I had to take the morning after pill.

Dr. M. asked me the same questions and recited information about the importance of consistently using condoms and the need to protect myself against sexually transmitted diseases. Dr. M. said I should use birth control if I couldn't be counted on to use condoms regularly.

As she talked, Dr. M. bobbed her head back and forth with the authority of a judge with her gavel, saying, "If you keep this up, it's only a matter of time before you get pregnant." I felt stupid having to listen to her speech. I hated feeling like I was a stereotype, one of too many black girls who can't remember to use condoms and end up pregnant.

Dr. M gave me the first of the pills right there in her office with instructions to take the next one in 12 hours. I took the last pill at 9:30 that night in the library, well on my way into studying all night.

They were the smallest pills in the world, but they felt larger than the vitamin horse pills I take daily. I felt hopeful that the worst was over when I swallowed the pill and said, "Now do your thing." Luckily, I didn't suffer any physical side effects from the pills. There could've been nausea, vomiting, vaginal spotting, and headaches.

My pregnancy problem was over, but I still had a lot of questions. Over the next few days, I tortured myself with conflicting thoughts about sex and relationships, and wondered if I'd ever be tempted not to use condoms again. And I questioned if I should just have serious relationships and give up booty calls.

What hit me hardest about the experience was that I let my desire for sex get the better of me. Instead of putting off sex when things weren't working, I got caught up in the heat of the moment. I still feel that sex is a beautiful thing; my desire's normal. I've resumed a healthy sex life. But I try to control the situations in which I have sex so I don't do foolish things.

Dante actually called me about a month after my pill drama. He talked to me like nothing had happened. I told him that I had to take emergency contraception. He sounded relieved that I wasn't pregnant.

My new partner and I have had sex a couple times, and he's as insistent about using condoms as I've become. Like me, he's scared of pregnancy and infections, and wants to maintain his peace of mind.

Looking back to that weekend with Dante, I was too antsy about having sex with him. Now I take my time, time to enjoy the moment and remember to be safe.

The author was in college when she wrote this story.

For more information on the morning after pill, see p. 291.

What if I'm Pregnant?

Even safer sex can be stressful

By Genevieve Santos

One evening in April, my close friend Samantha texted me.

"I need to talk to you," she wrote.

"What's up?" I typed back.

Samantha said that she'd had sex with her boyfriend. He'd used a condom and withdrew before he came. Still, Samantha felt nervous. She told some of her friends what had happened, and one of them told her she could be pregnant.

"If you have sex with a condom and it doesn't break, then you're fine," I wrote her. Thanks to the brochures I'd read on birth control, I knew that condoms had a high success rate if used correctly.

Samantha was reassured when I wrote her that it was very unlikely that she was pregnant. But my advice obviously wasn't enough since she called me the following morning. "Hello?" I answered in a drowsy state.

"I'm still worried that I might be pregnant," she said.

I thought Samantha was being unnecessarily anxious about the situation. I told her to ignore her friend's comment. I kept on repeating, "You used the condom and it didn't break." The chances of her being pregnant were quite small.

A lot of girls aren't ready for how they'll feel after having sex. Even those who know how to use protection to prevent pregnancy still experience anxiety just over the act of having sex.

I have friends who've had similar stressful experiences. My friend Janice always used protection when she had sex with her long-time boyfriend, but even a condom wasn't enough to keep her from worrying.

"I always think that even 0.00001% of sperm can get into me and get me pregnant," she once told me. "It's really scary to be so stressed about getting your period."

She and her boyfriend dealt with that stress by deciding to focus more on other alternatives to sexual intercourse, like just spending time with each other or foreplay. Foreplay can involve hugging, kissing, touching and rubbing, among other things.

I sympathized with Samantha and Janice because I'd had a pregnancy scare. But unlike them, I was scared because I'd had unprotected sex.

I was messing around with a boyfriend. Things got hot, and he entered me. But then he quickly withdrew without ejaculating, since neither of us had a condom. I thought I was pretty safe, even though girls can get pregnant from pre-cum (a fluid that comes out before ejaculation).

The possible consequences of my actions didn't hit me until weeks later, when I was late for my period. My cycle's usually irregular, but I couldn't help but think I might be pregnant.

Days went by slower than usual because I was constantly aware that my period was late. In my room, alone after a long day, I worried. My period still hadn't come. My imagination ran ahead. I started to think about how my boyfriend and I were too young to be parents, and imagined my father disowning me if I told him I was pregnant.

I told Samantha that if she was constantly worrying every time she had sex, then she shouldn't be having it.

I wondered if I should buy a pregnancy test. I confided in my older cousin, who has two kids, and she listened to me patiently. She told me to wait a few more days to see if my period came before taking any action.

But after almost two weeks, I didn't know what to do. One night, I broke down and cried. I wanted to take back those stupid few seconds of pleasure, because it wasn't worth my present anguish.

Finally, more than two weeks after it was due, my period came. I was so relieved. After that incident, I promised myself to never let a guy enter me unless he was wearing a condom.

Samantha sounded like she had far less to worry about than I had. I believed she was so anxious partly because she wasn't emotionally ready to have sex.

Being ready for sex means accepting that sex can be stressful.

If Samantha was constantly worrying every time she had sex, then I thought she shouldn't be having sex, which I told her during our phone conversation. I didn't think it was worth her time worrying for days on end over a few moments of pleasure.

Samantha agreed with me that sex wasn't worth the constant anxieties. She said she discussed the issue with her boyfriend, and he said he wouldn't mind taking a break from sex. So they decided to do the abstinence thing for now.

There are ways to ease anxiety about sex. It's important to get information about safer sex from trustworthy sources like Planned Parenthood. Another good source of information is a health teacher or social worker/guidance counselor in your school. They can also refer you to different clinics and health services available to youth. Once you feel more informed about ways to deal with having sex, it's easier to enjoy it when you're using condoms and other contraceptives.

But I've also learned that being ready for sex means accepting that sex can be stressful, whether it's safer or unsafe. So if you feel that you're not ready, that's perfectly fine. By practicing abstinence, you're at 0% risk of getting a sexually transmitted infection or getting pregnant.

Genevieve was 17 when she wrote this story.
She graduated high school and attended college.

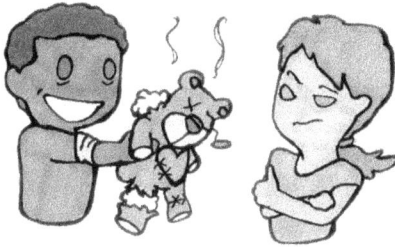

Chapter 3

Five Things to Ask About What Kind of Partner You Want

Do you know who you want to do it with?

If you're a virgin, you've probably had moments where you think everyone in the world has had sex—except you. You can't help but wonder what you're missing. Maybe you feel left out or just plain embarrassed when your friends talk about their sexual experiences and you have no stories to contribute. You start to ask yourself, "What am I waiting for?" Maybe you start to think, "Let me get it over with already."

But having sex shouldn't be just another item on your "to do" list. If you start to think about it like that, you're increasing the chance that your first experience won't be a good one. If you're single, you may find yourself doing it with someone you don't know very well or like very much, someone who

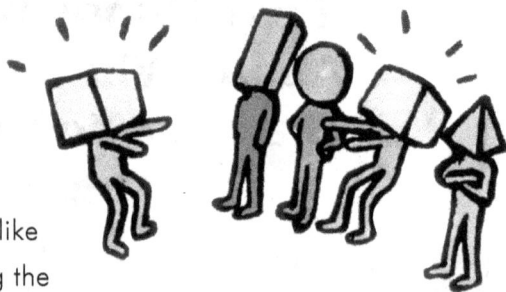

doesn't care enough about you to make sure they're making you feel good. And if you do it with someone you don't feel comfortable talking to, you're less likely to talk about—and use—contraception, too.

If you're thinking "I really want to have sex," and not "I really want to have sex with *this person*," remember that sex is not a generic experience that's the same no matter who you do it with. It can be awful or amazing, depending on who your partner is and how you feel about him or her.

Do you and your partner have similar expectations?

While you're thinking, "I'm really in love with this guy!" he could just be thinking, "Yeah, I want to hit that." While he's thinking, "This is the girl I want to be with forever," you could be thinking, "His friend is really cute."

No one wants to believe that their dream guy or girl just wants to hook up and move on, but it happens. On the other hand, you might think it's really clear that all you want is a one-night stand, but then you hear through the grapevine that the person you slept with was heartbroken you never called. Assuming that the other person wants exactly what you want is not a good idea, especially when the relationship turns sexual.

The best way to deal with this is to be up front about how you feel about the other person and what kind of relationship you want (or don't want) to have with her or him. If you're head over heels in love, you don't have to tell all your feelings the first time you hang out, or even the second or third. But if you're thinking of having sex and you still don't feel comfortable expressing how you really feel, ask yourself why. Is it because you're afraid to hear your partner's response? If you think express-ing your true feelings might mess up your rela-tionship—or your chance of having sex— you probably shouldn't be having sex with this person.

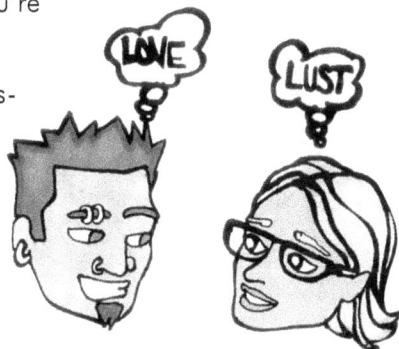

And if all you want is a one-night stand, be honest—even if it means that you might not get any.

Does your partner really care for you and make you feel special?

Some people find it pretty easy to say things like, "I love you," or, "You're the only one I want to be with." But when it comes to love, actions speak louder than words.

So ask yourself: Does your partner make you feel like you're really fun to be around? Do they express interest in the things you care about? Do they try to cheer you up when you're down or do little things that let you know they've been thinking about you even when you're not around? Do they make you feel like you can tell them anything? If you've answered "yes" to most of these questions, then you can be pretty sure that you're with someone who has real feelings for you.

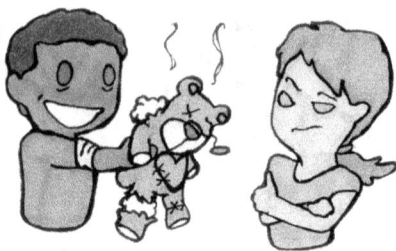

Someone who really cares is happy to see you and happy to hear your voice on the phone. They want to be seen in public with you. They call when they say they're going to call. They want to hear about your day and they notice when you're feeling blue.

If your partner says he (or she) cares, but his (or her) actions say something different, you might want to think twice—not just about sex—but about how good your partner is for you.

Even if you're thinking about having sex with someone you're not in a relationship with, sex always feels better with someone who respects you, protects you, and makes you feel good about you. If you are in a relationship, you should feel good about your relationship *before* you have sex. While sex can make a good relationship even better, sex, by itself, isn't going to make a bad relationship good.

Is your partner going out with anyone else? Are you?

Some people are capable of enjoying casual sex and some people aren't. If one of you is having sex with several different partners, while the other's life revolves around this one relationship, jealousy, resentment, and hurt feelings are bound to follow. Not to mention the fact that if either or both of you has other partners, your risk of STDs shoots up.

So be honest with your partner and with yourself. Don't pretend to be more—or less—serious about the relationship than you really are. If either or both of you is going out with other people, talk about that before taking your relationship to the next level.

Can you have a real and honest conversation with your partner?

Any couple that's been together happily for a long time can tell you that while sex is important, being able to talk to each other is more important. If you can't find anything to talk about, or don't feel comfortable bringing up the things you'd like to talk about, sex won't fill the void.

Even if you feel comfortable talking about everything under the sun, it still doesn't mean you should throw off your clothes and have sex. But if you can't talk, you definitely shouldn't. That's true whether or not you're in a committed relationship. After all, how are you going to make decisions about sex that feel comfortable to both of you if you can't talk to each other? And how will you handle it if something unexpected happens, like you lose your erection, or the condom breaks and you think you might be pregnant? Sex can be great, but it can also be messy. If you can't talk to your partner, you may end up dealing with some messy consequences alone.

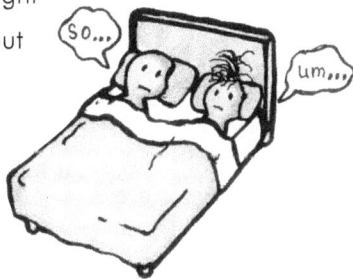

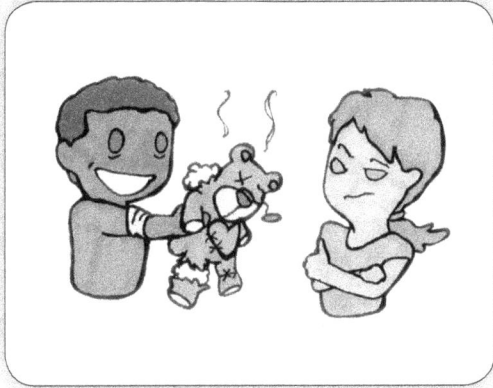

Looking for Love
Teens Share Their Experiences

Ready for Mr. Right

By Faleisha Escort

I had at least three boyfriends in high school. (I'm in my first year of college now.) I think the main reason I was attracted to these particular guys was the fact that they were easy.

Don't get me wrong, I liked them. But the main attraction was that they were easy prey! I already knew that they liked me, so I didn't have to work that hard to get them. They were my relationship guinea pigs.

None of these relationships lasted longer than a month or so, because I wasn't as serious as I thought I was, and neither were the guys.

The guys I went out with were always saying things like, "Oh, I want to be with my friends today," or, "I want to see this movie, not that one." I was just expected to sit back and have no opinions or objections.

I would go along for a while, doing what they wanted instead of what I wanted. But of course I got tired of that and ended the relationships. I felt disappointed and disenchanted.

The moment I realized I wanted a different kind of relationship came one night last summer when I was out with my (now ex-) boyfriend Derek (not his real name). We were at the movies, killing time, waiting for the show to start. So we went downstairs to the theater's little arcade section to chill. As soon as we got there, Derek headed toward the change machine and began popping quarters in one of the games.

At first, I'm like, "OK," since we were there and all, but then it got ridiculous. I was just standing there bored while Derek spent nearly half an hour pumping quarter after quarter into the machine. He must have gone through at least $5 worth of quarters! And get this: He has the same game at home.

I knew right then that I was going to break up with him after the movie. He made me feel less important to him than a video game. The fact that he was spending all this money combined with his lack of consideration for any of my feelings was the last straw.

Since becoming a free woman again, I've been thinking about what I want from my next relationship and how to go about getting it. This time I'm not going to settle for a guy who is easy to get.

The kind of guy who would immediately spark my interest is, of course, someone who I consider cute, or at least fair, in terms of looks. (Hey, looks aren't everything, but they do count!)

His intelligence level would be equal to mine. And his morals would give him self-respect and respect for the people he cares about. He would have had a spiritual upbringing. And he would love and respect his family and get along with them very well.

It's also important that the guy genuinely likes and cares about the same things I do. And he would not be the type who claims to want a monogamous relationship but can't seem to stop flirting with other female faces. I hate that.

This time I'm not going to settle for a guy who is easy to get.

Because I think you need to know all these things about a person before getting serious, I think a successful long-term relationship is most likely to stem from a strong, committed friendship. If you've developed love, trust, and mutual respect as friends and withstood the tests of disagreements, rumors, and other drama, then surely you are prepared to handle the not-so-different challenges of a romantic relationship.

I believe that if I develop a meaningful, long-term friendship with a guy I find to be both mentally and physically attractive, then I'd be able to move into a relationship more comfortably than with someone I barely know.

After making that transition from a long-term friendship to a romantic relationship, I think I would also feel more secure about the issue of sex (which will surely come up sooner or later).

I think the good thing about a long-term relationship with the right guy is the joy and security I would find in sharing my life fully and intimately with another person. It will be a challenge for me to be with the same person for months and years and still love him enough to not get tired of him. But that is the way I love my family and I would really like to experience that with a guy.

One day, I want to be able to say, "Gee, he knows me so well," and, just as important, "Wow, I know him so well." Am I ready for a long-term relationship? I don't know. But I am intrigued.

Faleisha was 18 when she wrote this story.
She went on to college, majoring in African-American Studies.

Nothing Like the Real Thing

Do guys want all of me, or just my body?

By Eric Green

Ever since I came out as gay, I've wondered, "Will I ever find me a man?" My friends tell me to wait and say it will happen "soon." But after some confusing experiences, I'm not even sure what I'm ready for.

My first relationship was with Eddie. I met him in 9th grade. We would read game magazines together at lunch and talk. Sometimes we cut class and left school early to go be alone together.

One day we were hanging out in the stairwell of his building, talking about video games and movies. Then Eddie asked me, "Do you have a sexual fantasy?"

"No, I don't have a sexual fantasy."

"You don't?! Everybody has a sexual fantasy."

"Well, I don't. I'm not the sexual type."

I could see where this was going and I was uncomfortable. We were sitting next to each other saying nothing. Then suddenly Eddie started to touch me and continued asking me sexual questions. I was nervous and kept thinking, "I'm not ready to have sex with him." But I also felt attracted to him and hoped that he could be my first boyfriend. So I fooled around with him.

After that day, Eddie and I kept fooling around. He would sweet-talk me, saying things like, "I like your body," and, "You're a great kisser." (True, I am a good kisser.) My friendship with Eddie meant a lot to me. I thought he was the perfect guy.

We were together for years, though, and during all that time we were never officially boyfriends. I finally confessed that I wanted to take it to another level. But I could see it in his eyes that he wasn't sure that he wanted to be my boyfriend.

Sure enough, he told me that he only liked me as a friend. I went home feeling broken-hearted. I felt that our years together did not mean much to him and that he played me for a fool. I got mad and did not want anything to do with him.

Soon after that, Eddie started dating my friend Carlos and I got very jealous. Luckily, it only lasted a few weeks, and Eddie and I eventually became friendly again.

Then I met Joe at the park. Joe was the same sign as me, Aquarius. He was 31 years old—too old for me—but he had a good personality. He would show up at the park on his bicycle, chatting with his friends. One day we were alone and Joe started flirting with me. I went into a store to buy soda and out of nowhere Joe came up and kissed me on my neck.

"What was that for?" I said.

"'Cause you're so sexy," he said. I wasn't sure that I should trust him. But I let him take me to a stairway where he started kissing me and caressing me. I was like, "What am I doing?"

Then he wanted me to give him oral sex. I had to make a quick decision. I refused. He got mad at me and said, "Someday, you'll know how good it feels."

"Whatever," I said. I was really uncomfortable.

I continued seeing Joe around, though, and I liked getting to know him as a friend. He was funny, and I looked for him at the park when I was there. But soon he started pressuring me for sex again.

"Hey, what's up?" Joe said one day. "How's school?"

"Oh, school's fine," I said, thinking, "I'm only in high school! This guy is bald. He's too old for me!"

"So what is up with you? Why are you playing me?"

"I'm not playing you," I said. "I am a very busy person. I am focusing on important things."

"So I'm not important?"

"I don't have time for relationships."

"Why do you have such an attitude?" Joe said.

"OK, I have to go now," I said, feeling confused.

Joe only wanted sex. He wasn't concerned about getting to know me; all he was concerned about was my looks. Plus, Joe is not real with himself. Once I asked him, "Are you gay?"

"No, I'm not gay! I just like to get my (bleep) sucked!" he said.

I thought, "If he is messing around with a gay person, that makes him gay, too."

I didn't know if he wanted a relationship or just wanted to try things out with a man.

I was glad I realized right away that he was only focused on having sex with me, and did not deserve my trust. Usually, though, it's more confusing whether someone wants to know me or just use me. Last year I went to visit my friends Nellie and Peter for the weekend. We were chatting and watching TV, smoking weed and eating chocolate chip cookies. Then Nellie left Peter and me alone. It grew silent for a few minutes. Peter crossed the room to sit by me and said, "Can you keep a secret?"

"Yes," I said, and Peter kissed me on the lips and then my neck. Chills ran up and down my spine and I was going with the flow until we got nervous that Nellie was coming back. Peter's secret was that he was bisexual.

I wanted to see him again after that, but I didn't know if he wanted a relationship or just to try things out with a man. Since then, we've continued fooling around, but I feel confused about where it's going.

I'm not the casual sex type. Some men are only about sex, and that's a total turn-off for me. I am more of a friendship kind of person. I get involved with guys and wonder, "Are these men in love with me or in love with my body?"

Recently, I had an experience that seemed like it would lead to having a real boyfriend. I started to get closer to my friend Carlos, who I've known for years.

I got locked out of my house late one night, so I spent the night with Carlos. We were talking and listening to the radio, writing poems and watching TV. Following that, we went to bed and slept next to each other.

I started to visit Carlos more and more, sometimes spending a few weeks at his house, staying up late, having private talks, and sleeping until mid-afternoon. It felt comfortable because Carlos was a close friend and he really knew me and liked me.

Then out of left field one day, he said, "I told Damion (another friend of ours) that I wanted to have sex with you."

I don't want to get attached to someone who will let me down.

His comment threw me off guard. All I could say was, "Oh, really?" We were sitting there staring at each other, saying nothing.

I felt awkward, like I was acting aloof and distant. I wondered, "Why don't I feel ready for this?" After all, Carlos is a good friend. I like getting his attention and I would not mind having sex with him.

But I realized that I am still very nervous about sex and who I have sex with. I don't want to become infected with anything, especially HIV, and I don't want to get attached to someone who will let me down.

Right now, I'm thinking that I should continue fooling around with the guys I really like, people like Peter and Carlos. They're not ashamed of who they are, and they understand that friendship comes first. But I'm going to wait for a relationship that really feels good to me, and I'm going to wait to have sex until I'm sure that a man is committed to me.

Eric was 21 when he wrote this story.

Me and Zarah... Zarah and Everyone Else

By Anonymous

Sometimes when you develop a deep passion for someone, you abandon the principles you've tried hard to hold onto. I discovered this the hard way through my relationship with Zarah.

I first saw Zarah in math class during my freshman year in high school. Then one afternoon during my sophomore year, I was waiting for the subway when Zarah and her friend Delilah saw me and said hi. We got on the train together and talked about school. The next day, I rode with them again. This time her other friend Daisy joined us. Soon, riding the train with them became routine.

Zarah and I lived far from each other, but she'd often ride to my stop and then turn around and go back home. One day I decided to keep Zarah company while she was waiting for the train back. About seven trains passed, but we couldn't break away from our conversation.

I revealed things that I normally don't tell people, like the time I stole money from my aunt. She told me about her rocky relationship with her mother and her wild years of junior high.

She also told me she was bisexual. I was a little shocked because she was always the first one to talk about a cute boy, or approach a guy and get his phone number. Still, I saw nothing wrong with her sexuality. I actually thought it was cool because now I could talk to her about girls, too.

After our disclosures, our subway conversations became routine. Zarah and I talked about topics ranging from the people she played to why the sky was blue. There were no dull moments or dead silences.

Chilling with Zarah was the highlight of my day.

Because of our subway talks, I sometimes got home two or three hours late and lied about where I was so that I wouldn't be grounded. She was getting in trouble too, so we switched to talking on the phone.

We sometimes spoke from 8:00 at night till 1 in the morning. I believe that if you can talk to someone for five hours, then you've really got something going on.

But Zarah and I didn't have anything going on romantically. As our friendship grew more intense over our sophomore year, people in school started asking if we were dating. We told some people that we were cousins in order to get them to stop bothering us.

But then I started questioning why I wasn't I going out with her, or at least why I hadn't tried to.

By late May, I noticed things about her physically that I'd overlooked before, like her "wow" body and her soothing brown eyes that made me space out and think of having a family.

Still, I felt hesitant about dating Zarah because she wasn't just any friend, but a best friend that I didn't want to lose. Plus, Zarah often told me about the boys and girls that she was dating or flirting with, and I didn't want to be just another person whom she was playing. To make matters more complicated, Zarah had a crush on Daisy, who had a boyfriend. And I had a gut feeling that Daisy liked Zarah too.

But by the summer, I couldn't hold a conversation with Zarah without thinking of how attractive she looked or how much I wanted to date her. My feelings were so strong that I needed to let them out. I figured I'd tell her, she'd turn me down, and then I'd move on. So one day in July I called her. Ten minutes into the conversation, I made my move.

"Um, Zarah, I kind of...um, well, I kind of like you."

She laughed.

"That's nice," she said. But "nice" wasn't what I was trying to get at.

"Well, um, do you like me?"

"I don't at the present time, but I possibly could," she replied.

I was taken aback. My plan to tell her just to get it off my chest and get rejected was foiled by a newfound possibility.

"So what do you want to do about it?" she asked. "Do you want to go out?"

"Well...um, I, I don't...I don't want to mess up our friendship."

I felt like a dumbass. She was intelligent, beautiful, and could make me fall out laughing. "Idiot! What the hell are you doing?" I thought.

But then I remembered that most of the relationships Zarah had were short-lived and that despite how close we were as friends, I feared ours would be the same. I valued her friendship immensely and didn't want to jeopardize it.

Zarah said that if our friendship was as strong as I thought it was, then it would last even if we dated, which almost convinced me. But then I remembered Daisy. I pictured me being with Zarah and her thinking about Daisy. So, despite Zarah's reassurance and my intense attraction, I decided to wait.

About two weeks after I told Zarah I liked her, I called her to see what she was up to.

"Guess what I did today?" she said, about to burst.

I took a wild guess. "You hung out with Daisy?" I asked.

"Yeah, and guess what else?"

"I don't know...what?"

"I slept with her!" she blurted. My jaw dropped and my fantasies of dating Zarah died like a slug in salt.

But Zarah had her fling with Daisy, then quickly lost interest in her. When Zarah told me that she was over Daisy, my feelings for her came out of hibernation. But over the course of several weeks, Zarah shuffled through more girlfriends.

Soon Zarah met a girl named Karen over the Internet, and they started dating. Karen was interesting, smart, funny—supposedly everything Zarah wanted in a girl's personality. But Zarah also thought Karen was overweight and didn't like the way she dressed, so Zarah's attraction to Karen fizzled.

That made me see flaws in Zarah. I felt that if she liked Karen's personality so much, it shouldn't matter whether she was overweight or unfashionable. I had a feeling that if we were to date, Zarah would find something wrong with me, or even cheat on me. How would I be different from the other people she played? Still, I couldn't let go of my visions of Zarah and me together.

By the beginning of our junior year, we were both so busy that we didn't talk or hang out as much as we used to. We became distant and that worried me, so I asked her if she wanted to hang out one weekend. We went shopping and then went to the Promenade, a nice park by the water in Brooklyn.

> **I didn't want a casual relationship, but I thought, "Something is better than nothing."**

The Promenade was nearly deserted. We sat on a bench and talked till the sun went down, and that's when, out of the blue, things got complicated. We didn't have sex, but I can tell you it was more physical than a kiss. To me, that moment was meaningful, because it was the first time I'd ever been so physical with a girl. And it was with Zarah.

But during our walk to the train station, there was a dead silence I'd never experienced with Zarah before. She put on her headphones. I wanted to talk about what happened and didn't understand why there was this uncomfortable hush between us.

After that, we didn't talk for weeks. When we finally did, I told her I regretted what we did because it's something I feel I should only do when I'm in a relationship with someone. As soon as I finished telling her how I felt, she skipped to another topic, and talked about this girl that she liked and a guy that liked her. I was hurt.

But I couldn't let it go. A week later, I had a new idea. I'd tell Zarah about the problems I was having with a "nameless" girl, who was actually her, and if she didn't figure it out, she'd give me the sort of advice that would work for herself.

So I told Zarah that I liked this girl but that she was involved with all these other people. She told me I should casually date the girl, which meant we'd be free to date others. When I revealed that the mystery girl was her, Zarah asked me if I wanted to "casually date" her.

I was unsure. I never got to see my parents together, so having a relationship with only one other person is important to me. Plus, emotional intimacy is what I want the most from a relationship.

Though I opened up to Zarah as a friend, I wasn't sure if I could do that romantically knowing she was also with someone else. I didn't want a "casual" relationship, but I'd been longing for Zarah for what seemed like forever. And I didn't want to be lonely.

I knew that whatever we did that was special to me, like kissing, she was doing with someone else.

So I thought, "Something is better than nothing" and told Zarah, "Yes." But even after we officially started dating, we hardly talked and made no advances in our relationship.

In my mind, I knew that whatever we did that was special to me, like kissing, she was doing with someone else. When I thought of her with other people, I felt like I was in a relay race rather than a relationship. I really liked Zarah and maybe even loved her, but I couldn't lie to myself and say that I was comfortable with our relationship.

The whole issue bothered me so much that two weeks into the relationship, I called her up to tell her that I couldn't do the casual dating thing. But she beat me to the punch.

Zarah said that Karen lost weight, so they decided to get back together. Zarah assured me that this time she intended to be faithful and wasn't going to see other people. My feeling that she'd drop me was right.

In the aftermath of the drama I went through with Zarah, I realized that I wanted her to be someone she clearly was not. She had many qualities I was attracted to, but I was looking for someone to settle down with and she wasn't that type of person. Because I couldn't accept that even though the evidence was clear, I ended up feeling regretful and disappointed.

Zarah and I are still friends, and sometimes I still catch myself dreaming that we're more than just friends. Then I remember all I've been through with her and wake up. Sometimes things are a certain way because they need to be. After seeing all the b.s. I went through just trying to talk to Zarah about us, I see that a serious romance probably would've been far worse.

The author was in high school when he wrote this story.

Messing Around Is No Match for Love

By Christian Galindo

I used to think that going out with many girls was cool. I think I got that idea from my cousin Jimmy. He's five years older than I am and I've always looked up to him. Jimmy was a "dog." He fooled around and slept with many girls, which made me think that's how guys naturally are.

When I was 13, I distinctly remember him telling me, "Chris, you shouldn't fall in love with any girl just like that. Play around. Enjoy your life." Jimmy said that getting serious with a girl would cause me problems. Although I was dating a little here and there when he told me this, I was mostly dedicated to my schoolwork and wasn't thinking about girls and relationships that much.

It wasn't until I turned 14 that I became really interested in the opposite sex. During the spring of 9th grade, I got involved with Jane. We messed around for about a week. About two months after I stopped seeing Jane, I met Kate. We hung out a lot and messed around, but to me it wasn't serious. I only told a few people in school that we were together because I still wanted to go out with other girls from school. Kate and I often argued about my refusal to commit to her. We stopped dating after a month and a half.

I was trying to follow Jimmy's advice by having fun and not complicating my life. Besides, the girls I'd messed around with were conceited. I didn't want to get seriously involved with a girl who had that type of personality.

Then, one day during the fall semester of 10th grade, I went up to my friend Angela in the hallway at school to say "hi." As she opened her locker, I noticed the girl next to her. She had the face of an angel.

"Christian, this is Paula," Angela said. "She's new in school."

Looking at Paula, I felt hypnotized.

"Nice to meet you, Christian," she said.

"Nice to meet you, too," I said. "I guess I'll be seeing you around." From then on, I stopped and talked to Paula whenever I saw her in the hallway. We soon became friends.

> **My cousin said that getting serious with a girl would cause me problems.**

I felt very attracted to Paula. She had a heavenly face and shapely body, but most important, she was down to earth and natural. She rarely wore makeup, preferring Chapstick to lipstick. She was friendly and helped people out, unlike some of the girls I'd gone out with.

I'd never gotten to know a girl like Paula before. I wanted to spend more time with her. I wanted to be her boyfriend. I felt like I had to disregard Jimmy's advice, because my heart told me I should be with her.

I told Angela that I liked Paula a lot. Angela said that Paula cared more about a guy's personality than his looks. Three months after we met, I asked Paula to be my girlfriend, hoping she liked my personality. She said she had to think about it. A week later, Paula told me she didn't want to be my girlfriend because she didn't know me well enough. I felt bad, because I liked her so much. But I accepted her decision.

Summer came and I still thought about Paula, but rarely saw her. When fall came around, I started to talk with her during my free time after school. Over the weeks, she became my best friend. I still wanted Paula to be with me, but didn't want to mess up the beautiful friendship we'd established.

When our school's Halloween dance came up, I invited Paula, just as a friend. But something was different that night. We were dancing in the middle of the darkened cafeteria. Red, green, and blue lights shone across Paula's face from a disco ball. The DJ put on a romantic, slow song. Suddenly, Paula hugged me. I was surprised, but I hugged her back. Then we kissed!

It didn't feel real. I thought I was dreaming. But then I realized that this meant she'd be my girlfriend. After we kissed, I asked Paula again to be my girlfriend, and she said "Yes." I was overjoyed.

Over the next few weeks, I discovered how good it was to have Paula be such a huge part of my life. Everyone in school soon knew we were a couple. We started cooking and doing homework together. I also introduced Paula to my mother and grandmother, which I'd never done with any of my previous girls.

But I was scared. I realized I was starting to fall in love with Paula, and I felt like I was showing her more love than she was showing me. I soon told her I was starting to fall in love with her and that I wanted to know if she felt the same way too. I told her I feared that she'd hurt me because she wouldn't care for me as much as I cared for her.

She said that I had to trust her. "I'm also falling in love with you," she said. "Let's just let time do its work." Her words were a relief. I agreed to see what would happen.

I was scared. I realized I was starting to fall in love with Paula.

I realized that being in a serious relationship is far more important to me than messing around. It has helped me to discover what love's about. If I hadn't already gotten to know Paula on a deeper level, I wouldn't be able to experience what it's like to trust my girlfriend and feel supported unconditionally. I feel much happier being so close to someone than when I was just messing around.

But we've also had conflicts. Paula can be very stubborn and often wants to do things her own way. In the past, when we had disagreements, she would keep arguing her points even when she knew I was right. I felt confused. I wanted to be with her, but felt like I'd start to resent her if I had to continue dealing with her attitude. I told her that if she kept being so stubborn, I'd prefer to break up. She said she'd try to change. And she has. She listens more to what I say and doesn't push her arguments as much as before.

We've also argued about the amount of time we spend together. I'm usually available on the weekends, which is when she has to do chores with her mother and complete her schoolwork. I get angry because I want to see her more, and my anger in turn makes her upset with me. But, even though I want to spend more time with her, I've come to realize that she has other responsibilities in her life. I know she's doing all she can to spend time with me, so I've resolved not to get angry with her over that issue anymore, particularly since I'm only spoiling our quality time. We communicate well with each other, which helps us get over our conflicts. So far, we've been together for six months.

I care a lot about Paula, as much as I care for myself, and sometimes even more than that. When she's sick, I wish I could be sick in her place. I never thought that I could love someone so much. I know some guys will still say that being a player is the best way to be. But I know that, for me, messing around is no match for being in love.

Christian was 16 when he wrote this story.

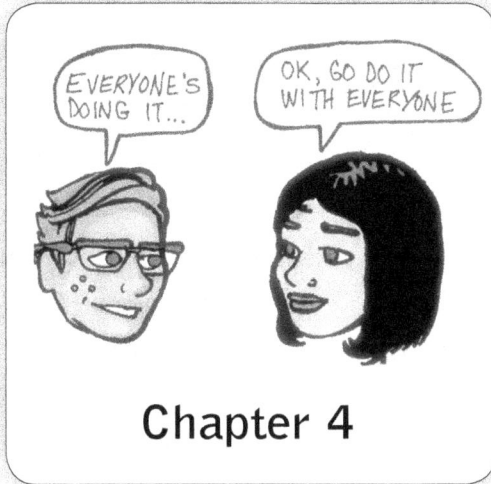

Six Things to Ask
to Make Sure Your Partner
Isn't Mr. or Ms. Wrong

Are you pretty close to the same age?

Let's face it: a 25-year-old, even a 20-year-old, has more experience and can do more things in the world than a 15-year-old. Healthy sexual relationships involve mutual respect and a lot of give-and-take. When there's a big age difference, it's hard to have an equal relationship. The older person tends to dominate and that's usually not a good thing for the younger person. The younger person may end up doing things, sexually and otherwise, that she (or he) doesn't really want to do. In general, if you're the younger person, you may find it hard to just be yourself because you're worried about doing or saying something that your older partner will think is immature or unsophisticated.

That doesn't mean younger and older people can't be attracted to each other or don't get crushes on each other. They do, all the time. But acting on those crushes is usually not a good idea.

Has your partner ever pressured you to do something that made you uncomfortable?

It could be anything from lying to your parents to doing drugs to having sex before you're ready. Asking you if you want to do something or try something is one thing. Continuing to push you to do it after you've said you don't want to is something else. A partner who pressures you is showing you that he or she is more interested in pleasing him or herself than in making you happy. If the person you're with is being that selfish, you may want to rethink the relationship.

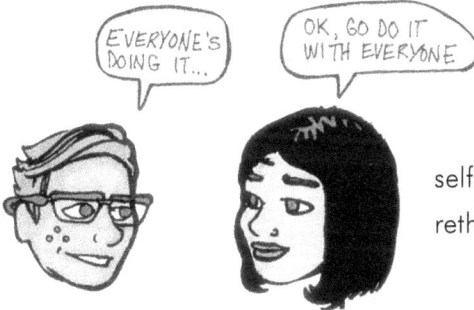

Do you feel safe with your partner?

If you feel safe around your partner, that's good. It means you trust him or her. If that's the case, you might feel comfortable having sex with them.

But if your partner has ever done anything that scared you, think hard before you take your relationship to the next level. They may have gotten really angry over something small, yelled at you or hit you, or threatened to hurt you or himself/herself.

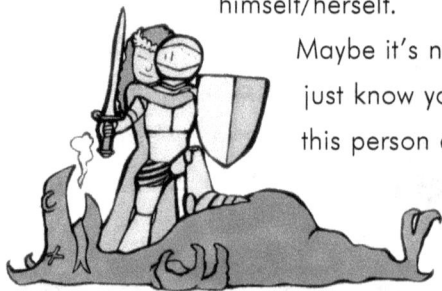

Maybe it's not even that clear-cut—you just know you feel on-edge around this person and you aren't sure why. That feeling is more than enough reason not to get involved. Trust your gut if you feel unsafe with someone and break it off.

It's also important for you to know that abusive relationships tend to follow a pattern. After hitting or otherwise hurting their partners, abusers will usually act as if they're really sorry for what they did. They'll apologize profusely, treat you really nicely, maybe buy you presents, and promise to never, ever do it again. But they almost always do—hurt you again, that is.

If you stay with an abusive partner because he convinces you that he "didn't really mean it," chances are you'll find yourself caught in a truly vicious cycle. As time passes, the "honeymoon" periods of good behavior get shorter and the incidents of violence get more frequent. Don't let yourself get caught in that cycle.

Is your partner too controlling?

Abusive relationships usually develop gradually. There are warning signs that come before physical violence. One of the most common is overly controlling behavior.

If your partner tries to tell you what you can wear, where you can go, and who you can hang out with, that's overly controlling.

If your partner is so jealous and distrustful that he's always checking up on you, wanting to know where you are and who you're with every minute of the day, that's overly controlling.

If your partner tries to isolate you from other people, coming between you and your family or close friends, or makes you feel like you have to choose between him and other things in your life that are important to you, that's overly controlling. Physical abuse can follow.

If you don't do exactly what he says, your partner will use that as an excuse to punish you. The abusive partner will even try to convince you that his behavior is your fault—if you acted right, he'll say, he wouldn't have to hit you. Don't fall for it.

Sometimes people mistake overly controlling behavior for love. It's easy to be flattered when someone seems so intensely interested in you, especially at first. You might think, "He loves me so much, he wants me to be with him all the time and he can't bear to have me think about anything but him." But someone who tries to prevent you from having a life outside of your relationship with him, who tries to take away your independence, or who says you can only be together if you do things his way, doesn't really love you.

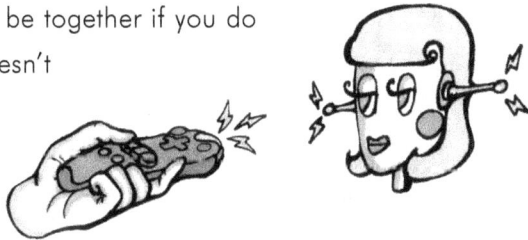

Are you uncomfortable introducing him or her to your family and friends?

Sometimes there's a good reason to keep a relationship you're involved in a secret. If you're gay and are sure your parents would freak out if they knew, you're probably not going to be introducing them to your sweetie. Likewise, if you know your parents are prejudiced against people of a particular group and the person you're seeing happens to be one of *them*, you're probably going to hesitate before bringing your special someone home.

But there are probably other people in your life—friends, siblings—that you can talk to about the relationship. They can help make your boyfriend or girlfriend feel accepted and welcome rather than a dirty secret.

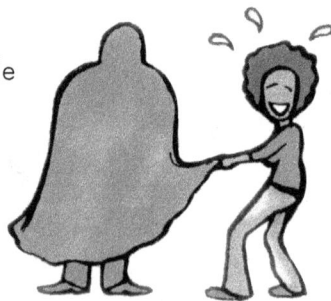

If a relationship is going well and makes you happy, you usually want to show it off. So when you make an effort to hide a relationship, to keep it separate from the rest of your life, you need to stop and ask why. Is there something about the person you're seeing or how the relationship is going that makes you uncomfortable or is causing you pain? Something that would embarrass or shame you in front of the other people you care about? Would friends and family have a legitimate reason to be concerned if they knew about your relationship? For example, are you going out with someone who is either a lot older or a lot younger than you are; is disrespectful or abusive toward you; or is involved in something that could end up getting you both in trouble (like drugs or gangs)?

Whatever your doubts are, feeling like you have to keep your relationship secret is a warning sign that something's not right.

Have you ever been in an abusive relationship or been sexually abused?

If you've been abused, it can have a long-term effect on your future relationships. For example, survivors of sexual or relationship abuse sometimes have a hard time judging whether a new partner will keep them safe. They may put themselves in dangerous situations without realizing it, and risk being abused again. Other victims seek relationships where they can be in control, and end up abusing others. They may become promiscuous, or avoid intimate relationships altogether.

This does *not* mean that everyone who's been abused is doomed to be alone or mistreated. It does mean that you should be careful. It's important to talk about what happened to you, even if it happened a long time ago, so you can process your feelings and be aware of how the past may still be affecting you. The best way to do this is in therapy. (See p. 312 for information on finding free or low-cost counseling and support groups near you.)

It's also important to be extra careful about who you get involved with. When you're getting to know someone new, take it slow. Be alert to things that make you uncomfortable, and take your feelings seriously. Ask yourself the questions in this book. And talk to people you trust—friends, parents or other family members, teachers, or counselors—to help you figure out if a relationship is safe for you.

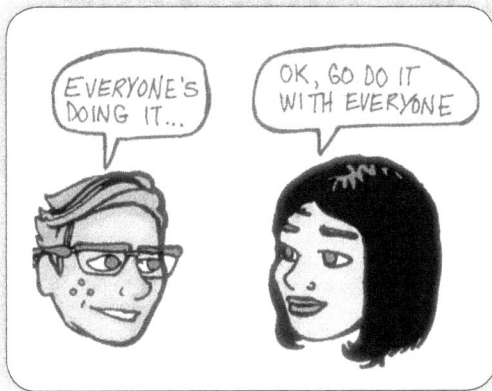

What to Watch Out For
Teens Share Their Experiences

Younger Girls/Older Guys

By Anonymous

Many girls, including myself, are attracted to older guys because they seem more mature than guys our age.

Many boys still in high school tend to look sloppy, as if they don't care about anyone or anything. That's not appealing. And guys out of high school tend to have jobs, and money to buy their girls gifts and to take them places. I don't want to have a guy ask me to go to a movie and then ask me to pay for it myself. My friends and I feel that for that, we can go out with our friends and not worry about the pressure of being on a date.

Some girls I know like the "show and tell" of being with an older guy. They like to walk around their friends with their "man," then talk about him with their friends when he leaves. They talk about how cute he is and what he gives them or doesn't give them. They rate his sexual performance or, if they're not having sex, his kissing skills. I guess some girls show off guys their own age as well, but I've never seen a girl show off her "boy."

I've been with two guys who were more than three years older than I was. I met Tony when I was 15 and he was 19. More recently, I went out with Bobby, who I met through friends in the neighborhood. He's 25—eight years older than I am.

I've heard some people say that girls who go with older guys are looking for a father figure. Maybe that's true in my case, because I was raised with no father and have no brothers. And though I'm a strong-willed person, I sometimes like it when my man tells me what to do, like when to go home and how to dress. If what he wants me to wear is too expensive, though, I also want him to buy me clothes.

I'm OK with wanting a control freak as long as he's not abusive when I don't do what he wants. I guess I'm impressed if someone can both show he's mad at me and control his anger by not becoming physical.

I'm not sure why I don't want to have more power in my relationships with guys. I guess it's because being controlled makes me feel cared for. I think I'd feel weird if a guy asked me what I wanted to do or where I wanted to go, because I've never dealt with a guy who wasn't controlling. A younger guy could try to tell me what to do but my feeling about that is, "How's he gonna control me if he's controlled by his mother?"

But telling me what to do isn't the only thing a guy can do to make me feel cared for. If a guy shows interest in talking to me, rather than just sleeping with me, then that also makes me feel he cares for me.

And sometimes guys can get carried away with bossy behavior. Bobby, the oldest guy I've been with, wanted to know where I was and what I was doing when I wasn't with him. At first, I was impressed by his interest and felt that he must really care about me. But he was soon acting like that all the time, and it started to bother me. That's one of the reasons we're not going out anymore.

I'm attracted to older guys, but sometimes the age difference leads to different expectations about the relationship.

Even though I'm attracted to older guys because I think of them as more mature, sometimes the age difference leads to different expectations about the relationship. Bobby also talked a lot about having a family with me. He was ready to settle down, but I wasn't ready for that.

And sometimes older guys don't act any more mature than younger guys. My friend Sandra is also into older guys. A year ago, when she was 15, an 18-year-old guy who sold drugs on her block began to talk to her every night before she went home. She said she was attracted to him because he had game. "Something about the way he walked," she said. He was bad and the both of them knew it.

When they started going out, she liked being known as his girl. But he never took her anywhere, and that bothered her. There goes the idea that an older guy will take a girl out. I had that problem with Tony, too. I felt that he was embarrassed to be seen with me, perhaps because I was too young.

Now Sandra's man is in jail and he expects her to wait for him. But that's not her plan. Now that she's 16, she shows some interest in guys her own age as well as those older than she is. I noticed in my friend's case that an older guy may be a smoother talker and dress better, but that doesn't mean he'll have much respect for the younger girl he goes out with.

Even though my friends and I prefer older guys, we also need to remember that just because they're older, it doesn't mean they'll act more mature or more grown-up. And if a guy's too embarrassed to be seen with his girl because she looks too young, then he should find a girl his own age.

The author was 17 when she wrote this story.

Looking for Maturity

By Anonymous

I've only had three boyfriends. My first, Leap, was the same age as I was. We met when we were 16. Leap went to an all-boys school and I met him at one of his school's parties. He called me and we got to know each other.

Everything was nice in the beginning. Simple things he did impressed me, like meeting me at my school or giving me cards with cheesy poems signed "Love, Leap." We also went to movies.

But we didn't have any deep conversations. I didn't want to talk about basketball statistics and hip-hop lyrics, or sit through some stupid movie. If I suggested something different, like a movie that didn't contain slapstick and farting, he acted as if I was suggesting we do something outrageous.

Other things I found interesting struck him as ho-hum or difficult. Sometimes I felt like I had to dumb myself down just for the sake of our conversations.

After my relationship with Leap, I became increasingly disgusted with how boys my age acted. I would see them standing around, not doing anything but cracking jokes on people who passed by.

While waiting in line at one party I went to, I couldn't believe how rowdy a group of guys were acting. They were jumping on cars, drinking cheap liquor—just acting stupid. The party was almost canceled because they wouldn't calm down.

I'm not saying that all 16- and 17-year-old guys act stupid and immature, but at the time, that's all I saw. I even began to feel like I was acting too old or stuck up.

Then I met a tall, bulky guy named Pablo. He approached me and told me that he remembered seeing me around the neighborhood. We started to talk. I liked the way he spoke, so I had no problem giving him my number.

When Pablo told me on the phone he was 22, I was surprised. I'd thought that he was my age, just with some sense. I was hesitant to start dating him because he was six years my senior. I thought he might try to take advantage of me because of my age. Or that he thought I'd get with him because he could buy me things I couldn't afford. Or that he only wanted sex.

Despite my reservations, we went out to the movies. Later, we talked about college, our plans for the future, and other subjects Leap never touched on. I was so happy I was able to talk to him without him saying something I considered dumb.

We began to date, and in the beginning, everything was fine. He always returned my calls, unlike Leap, and he took me out to dinner at nice restaurants, not pizza places. Pablo made more money than Leap, and Leap just didn't know much about anything outside of his neighborhood.

But about four months into the relationship, Pablo became very mistrustful of me. He scanned numbers in my cell phone and questioned me about numbers with male names. He constantly called me to make sure I was where I said I'd be.

He didn't even like me to be around my friends, because he said that they were nosy and never liked him. My friends were skeptical of Pablo's intentions, but they weren't around him enough that he should've been so sure they were against him.

"Why is it that every time I see you, you have to look in my phone?

All the incoming calls are from you," I asked him.

"Well, if you don't have anything to hide, then it shouldn't bother you," he said. So I didn't say anything, even though it did bother me that he was constantly trying to catch me doing something wrong. He'd say things like, "Yeah, I gotta watch out for all those young guys outside your school."

I felt like walking around or going shopping with my friends was in some way wrong. When I did go with them somewhere, I didn't tell him because I knew it would turn into a huge argument.

After a year together, I ended our relationship because he couldn't trust me. After our breakup, I decided that I had let him take advantage of me by being afraid to tell him how much I disliked his insecurities. I wondered if I listened to and put up with him because he was older.

I didn't want to talk about basketball statistics and hip-hop lyrics, or sit through some stupid movie.

I met my next boyfriend, Jay, a month later at the Gap. I figured Jay was 18, but he turned out to be 22. His age made me hesitate, particularly after Pablo. I knew any guy could be jealous, but I felt that older guys are more likely to be jealous so I'm still cautious about Jay. I don't want to let things that bother me go like I did with my ex.

Sometimes I feel as if I'm boring Jay when I talk about prom or graduation. When I ask him if he's bored, he says he isn't, but just doesn't have the same level of excitement I have about those things. He's past that point in his life, so what's exciting for me is "been there, done that" for him.

But we've been together for two months. Jay seems a little more my speed. Even though he's older than I am, he seems to be more relaxed than Pablo and not as crazy as other guys.

Even though my current boyfriend is older than I am, older guys aren't my preference. I simply prefer someone I can relate to and who can relate to me. If I found a guy my age who I could relate and talk to, then there'd be no problem.

I know, sooner or later, I'll be around guys my age who I'll like. I suspect this will probably happen in college, because there I'll be in classes with guys who have the same interests as I do.

The author was in high school when she wrote this story.

I Paid a High Price for Love

By Anonymous

I was standing on the lunch line at my junior high school one day when I felt someone tug on my ponytail. When I turned around, a tall guy with short black hair was smiling slyly. I turned to my best friend and giggled. Then he did it again. I thought it was the cutest thing in the world. After we got our lunch, he sat at my table, but didn't say a word.

In French class, my friend Julie informed me that the guy with no vocal cords was named Danny. He was 15 and he wanted to go out with me, she said. "I don't even know the guy," I said with a laugh. Julie smiled and said, "Look, just get to know him. If you don't like him, you can dump him."

Danny followed me around to all my classes for the rest of the day but he didn't speak to me until after school, when he asked if he could walk me home. I told him he could. On the way, we stopped at the park and hung out for a while. We talked about our families, school, and music.

Danny had a sense of humor and made me laugh a lot. He seemed like a sweet guy. He was interested in everything I talked about and that made me feel special. I decided to go out with him.

I began spending time with Danny every day. We went to school together and hung out afterwards. He never failed to walk me all the way home. I felt like I could depend on him, and I needed someone to depend on.

Before meeting Danny, I was never happy with my life. My mother was always putting me down, making me feel worthless. I was yearning for someone to really love me and Danny became that person. I could talk to him about my problems at home. He would hold me when I was feeling down and promise that whatever happened, he'd be there. Because he made me feel safe and secure, I clung to Danny. I thought I'd found my savior. It took me a long time to find out how wrong I was.

One day, about three months into our relationship, I was wearing a bodysuit that I had just bought. When Danny saw me, he said, "You're my girl. Why do you want to wear that and show everyone what you have? Do you want to look like a slut?" He handed me his hooded sweater and said, "Put this on and zipper it." He made me feel ashamed of how I was dressed, even though everyone was wearing bodysuits at the time.

I put on the sweater and zipped it part way up. Danny wasn't satisfied; he zipped it up to my neck. He looked me in the eyes and said, "I'm going to check on you, so don't even think about taking it off." I thought this was his way of showing affection. I thought it was cute.

After that, Danny was constantly telling me not to do things. I couldn't wear makeup, skirts, or anything that he considered "slutty." I couldn't listen to a band I liked because he thought they played "devil music." I couldn't go to the store. I couldn't even hang out with my two best friends. Danny started cutting his classes to "check on me" and make sure I was doing what he said.

Danny justified giving me orders by making it clear that I was his property. "You're my girl," he kept telling me. And because I was his girl, I was supposed to listen to whatever he said. I didn't question this because I thought I'd be lost without him. At first, I didn't even notice how much he was controlling me. All I needed was for him to hold me. As long as his arms were tightly around me, I got what I wanted out of the relationship. With him by my side I was able to ignore my problems at home.

But, if I didn't do what he said, Danny would get angry—not just annoyed, but violently angry. As much as I hated admitting it, I was scared. I knew Danny had a short fuse and I didn't want to set him off. I was afraid of his temper but I was also afraid of losing him. So I obeyed him when he told me what to wear, to stay home if he wasn't with me and to ignore all my friends.

One day, about a year after I started going out with Danny, he wanted me to walk to his house, a mile and a half away. Because it was a freezing cold, snowy day, I said no. That was the first time I refused to do what he said.

Danny gripped my arm, twisted it to where it was painful, and pulled me. We were standing outside in my neighborhood and some people were out shoveling their sidewalks. I said no again in a firm tone, but low enough so that no one else could hear me. He twisted my arm more. With his other hand, he grabbed some of my hair and yanked me forward. Tears were forming in my eyes. I realized that the more I resisted, the more hurt I'd get and the more the neighbors would notice, so I tramped through the snow to his house.

I figured that once we got there, he'd leave me alone since he'd gotten his way. I was wrong. I didn't even have a chance to get my coat off before he punched me. Danny hit me everywhere except my face (knowing that would leave visible marks). He did slap my face once though, which demeaned me completely. Then Danny shoved me into a chair and forced off my shoes.

Danny justified giving me orders by making it clear that I was his property. "You're my girl," he kept telling me.

I began crying hysterically. The only person who cared for me (or so I believed) was treating me like I was nothing. Danny tossed my shoes on the top of a cupboard where I couldn't get to them. "Shut up," he said. "Take your coat off, you ain't goin' nowhere." I just sat there sobbing.

After about an hour of giving me dirty looks, Danny started to feel bad and apologized for everything. "I just wanted to be with you," he said. We made up. A couple of hours later, he got me my shoes and I went home like nothing had happened.

That type of incident became an everyday thing. I never said anything to anyone because I thought I deserved it. I believed Danny when he told me things like, "I'm the only guy who'll take your crap." And I figured that having Danny hit me was the price I had to pay for having him hold me.

I became more and more isolated. Danny would only let me see my friends when he was there. Since he had no problem hitting me in public and I didn't want my friends to see that, I avoided them. I was too depressed to even talk to them about what was happening. I knew they would feel bad for me and try to get me to leave him. Part of me wanted to but I dreaded being alone.

I did threaten to leave Danny a few times. His response was, "You can't get anyone else. Who would want you?" I believed him. I figured I would end up marrying him, dropping out of school and becoming a lonely, beaten-up housewife.

> **I figured that having Danny hit me was the price I had to pay for having him hold me.**

Things kept getting worse. One day, I was in the bathroom at Danny's house, combing my hair, getting ready to go out. I could hear him telling his sister and his cousin about a fight we had at a party. He had dragged me down a flight of stairs because I wanted to talk to someone other than him. But Danny told his sister he did it because I was a bitch.

From the bathroom, I yelled out, "You're such a liar!" Danny stormed in and pushed me hard enough to make me fall. I almost banged my skull on the bathtub. His sister started screaming, "I'm telling Mommy. I'm callin' the cops!" His mom came in with a bat, and started swinging it at him. She turned to me and said, "Don't worry, I'm sending him to live with his father." Danny ran out.

I was so incredibly embarrassed. At the time, I wouldn't have cared if he had killed me, but why did he have to do it in front of everyone? Danny's cousin was crying. She told me that he had grown up seeing his dad hit his mom. She begged me to leave him. "He'll never change," she said.

The cops arrived but Danny was gone. His family was out in the hall and I had to walk past them to leave the house. They stared at me pityingly. The police drove me home. That was the worst of all the times Danny hurt me because his entire family and the cops were involved. Everyone knew what was going on. Everyone wanted to protect me from Danny, when I thought Danny was my only protection.

For about four days after that, I tried to stay away from him. He would call me up and come to my house crying. I tried ignoring the phone and the doorbell. I wanted badly to go out and see my friends, but when I did, Danny was there, a puppy-dog look on his face. "I'll change," he said. "I promise. I'm sorry." I gave in...again.

I learned that the worst thing you can do to yourself is to depend completely on someone else.

I still believed Danny loved me. "He will change," I thought. But it was more like a hope. Sometimes hope just isn't enough. He never changed the way I wanted him to. He only got worse. I took his abuse for another five months, until his mother finally sent him away to live with his father. At last, I was free.

I was lucky. I didn't have to break up with him. His mom took care of the dirty work. Looking back, I blame myself for what happened. I should've stopped the vicious cycle sooner. I guess I was just terrified of being alone again. I was stuck in a pit of self-pity. Not even a slap in the face could wake me up.

For the first few months after Danny left, I didn't care what happened to me. I reunited with my friends but pretty much all we did was party. Then I met Greg. Neither of us was ready to jump into a committed relationship at first, so instead we became wonderful friends.

Greg made me realize that Danny wasn't the only person who could care for me. Greg not only cared; he supported me in a positive way. He insisted that I deserved a lot more than what I had. Greg somehow made me see that I had the power to accomplish anything. We started going out and have been together for two years now.

Writing this story has been the final healing phase for me. I am a different person now than I was when I was with Danny. Although it was a horrible experience, at least I learned a lesson from my relationship with him: The worst thing you can do to yourself is to depend completely on someone else. I will never do that again and I will never let anyone else control, abuse, or hurt me. I know now that you don't have to put up with that kind of treatment in order to be loved.

The author was in high school when she wrote this story.

Haunted by My Past

By Anonymous

After about a year of dating my boyfriend, Kevin, I began to have frightening flashbacks of the sexual abuse I experienced as a child. Since the flashbacks started, I've been uncomfortable having sex with Kevin. I've even started feeling threatened and victimized, the way I felt as a child, even though Kevin is not abusive toward me.

I never truly enjoyed sex, but after the flashbacks began I started to feel as if I wasn't even in the room anymore. I felt like a doll being rocked back and forth in a cradle while Kevin had sex with me. It reminded me of my father molesting me as a child.

I wanted to tell Kevin, or stop having sex with him, but I was afraid he wouldn't understand. In order to ignore my complicated feelings, I went back to the trick that kept me sane during the abuse: I detached my mind from my body.

I would tune in to the first time we met when he was just another face and remember how, after five years, he started showing interest in me and we began dating. I would romance about our relationship in my mind as if everything was going great between us, just to get through.

I don't know if the flashbacks led us to have problems, or if I started having the flashbacks because we were already in conflict. Whatever the case, we were having conflicts about control, and for me to be able to stand having sex, I have to be in control.

It's been six years since the judge granted me an order of protection from my father, but any reminder of his presence still alarms me.

Memories of the abuse he put me through haunt me.

Sometimes I get nightmares and wake up in a cold sweat in the middle of the night, or I get flashbacks when I'm in the shower or when I'm rubbing lotion against my skin. I feel really nervous and uncomfortable touching myself in even these minor ways because painful memories come back.

I remember one dreary evening waking up to the heavy scent of tobacco (my father was a smoker), though no one was in the house at the time. I felt his presence nearby.

My skin began to crawl and horrible feelings of my father depriving me of my childhood tormented me all over again. I cried, holding my underwear tightly against my skin. I wanted my virginity back.

I hated him for abusing his role as a father. He was supposed to be a male figure that I could trust and turn to. I hated my sexuality. I was angry at the world for what had happened to me.

When I became a teenager, memories of the abuse led me to grow protective of my body. I hated getting attention from men. I kept myself covered up to avoid any boys piercing their eyes at me.

When shopping for clothes, I made sure that nothing I bought was too revealing. No v-neck blouses, spaghetti straps, halter tops, or short skirts. I would be the only fool wearing a black denim jacket while roasting in 90 degree weather. I feared that by attracting attention from men I would be putting myself in danger. I was very cautious about the message I was sending.

When Kevin and I started dating, he was shy and very respectful. I'd never met anyone like him before. It took him months to have the courage to kiss me.

He also gave me full control over our relationship, which was something I wasn't always used to. At times I would yell at him just because I could, and he would start crying. He'd get worried when he did things to upset me. I smiled at this advantage behind closed doors. It felt good playing the dominant role in a relationship. I teased him and made him feel guilty if I didn't get my way.

I did these things because a part of me wanted revenge. I felt every man deserved the mighty strike of a woman's wrath. All my life I'd been surrounded by male figures like my father and uncles who would physically and sexually abuse and control their wives and, in my father's case, his children, too.

Eventually, Kevin caught on to the idea that I was taking advantage of him and grew tired of me always having things my way. He wanted me to stop walking all over him, so he started to yell and argue with me. But I was so fearful of losing control that I was willing to fight for my advantage.

Many times when I felt Kevin was trying to take over, I would get nervous and show off by proving to him who was boss. When I yelled at Kevin, I was yelling at him and my father—any man who tried to manipulate me.

It felt good playing the dominant role in a relationship. A part of me wanted revenge.

Soon we were arguing non-stop. On the phone, especially, we exchanged curses and insults. Sometimes he'd just explode in the street, yelling as if I was deaf. One time he ended up breaking his cellular phone in half because he was so angry with me.

Deep down we were both trying to prove something to one another. Kevin was also in foster care, abandoned by his mother, and our relationship probably raised fears in him, too, that neither one of us could understand. We were driving each other nuts.

Without feeling in control of our relationship, I could no longer feel comfortable having sex. But I didn't tell Kevin because I didn't think he would ever understand. I wasn't even sure that I understood what I was feeling.

I especially didn't want him to feel uneasy and worried around me, or to feel like I was accusing him of abusing me. I just wanted our relationship to feel the way it used to. I figured that my feelings would soon pass. Unfortunately, they didn't.

I felt like a victim, taunted by my past. I hated feeling that way. Trying to hide how I felt, I sometimes ended up drinking to make it easier for me to not feel ashamed of doing things I didn't want to do. Then, after a while, I started to feel like I didn't care anymore about how I felt. I found myself saying, "All that matters is that Kevin loves me."

I wasn't sure what was going on with me. I had no grip. I'd lost the control I had longed for. And what had happened to my values and my self-esteem?

Plenty of times I wanted out, but I felt I'd be lost without him in my life. At around that time, my sister and grandmother were both hospitalized for mental illness, and I was moved into a strange new foster home where no one cared about me and I had little contact with family or friends. I felt vulnerable and lonely. Kevin kept me company and gave me support. But with no one else to lean on, I grew too dependent on him.

I thought to myself, "Can Kevin and I find a way to be together without our pasts getting in the way?"

I tried to be careful of the things I said around him to avoid the arguments, but sometimes I felt I had no choice but to go off. I told myself, "I refuse to repeat my childhood and accept disrespect from anyone."

I guess Kevin felt the same way. He was just as concerned about getting his point across.

After two years, he announced that he wanted "a break." As much as I'd often longed for the same thing, I was furious and desperate. I spent hours over the phone trying to convince him to come back, but my pleas weren't enough.

After several days, I figured I would win Kevin back by having sex with him again. That night, we both ended up drinking heavily—maybe because we both felt uncomfortable—and had sex. I felt miserable afterwards because Kevin didn't immediately want to get back together. He said he still had feelings for me but the arguments were too much for him.

We decided to try to work things out, but to take things a bit more slowly. We both want to rebuild our trust in each other and stop fighting for control. I would like Kevin to be more considerate of my feelings and to understand that it hasn't been easy coping with my past experience, and I would like to be able to do the same for him.

I'm trying hard to separate the past from the present. Kevin isn't my father. Though we argue, Kevin does not intend to do harm to me. I need to stop exploding at every argument we have. Kevin and I have been together for a long time, and I'm hopeful that we can both be more understanding and patient.

I'm trying hard to separate the past from the present. Kevin isn't my father.

Lately, Kevin and I have been doing a lot of talking and hanging out and going to the movies. We've found lots of other activities to do together rather than have sex. I enjoy the time we're spending together because we're learning more new things about one another, and I don't have to feel pressure to have sex. I'm happy with the way things are now. I would like our relationship to remain this way until I feel ready for sex.

I am aware that it may be a long time until I can recover from the abuse I went through. But I can also see how far I've come. I used to fear and hate all men. Now I date and socialize with them. I am learning that some men, including Kevin, can be trusted.

I have to stop taking my anger out on Kevin, and I have to try not to control him. I hope he can do the same for me.

The author was 19 when she wrote this story.
She later attended college to study social work.

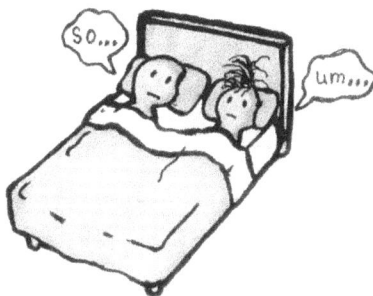

Chapter 5

Five Things to Ask About Intimacy

Do you know your partner's favorite color?

OK, you don't really *need* to know your partner's favorite color to be ready to have sex with him or her. Just like you don't need to know the music they like to listen to, the kinds of books or movies they enjoy, or their favorite food. But think about it: if you don't know the little things about your partner, how many truly important things are you also clueless about?

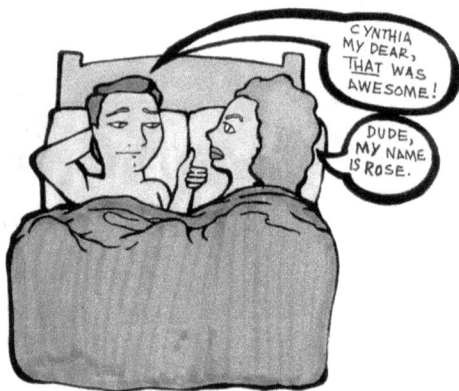

Have you and your partner ever had a fight? How did you resolve it and make up?

What does fighting have to do with sex? Think about it. People who always have to win an argument may also be determined about getting their own way in bed. People who always give in may show you a good time, but sooner or later they're sure to start feeling frustrated and angry and those bad feelings are going to come out. And someone who resorts to violence...well, that's scary enough when you're fully dressed and there are other people around. Imagine what it would be like if you were naked and alone together.

All couples fight sometimes. It's *how* you fight, and how you make up, that's important. Can you talk calmly about your disagreements? Can you can stand up for your point of view and find ways to compromise that are fair to both of you? Do you avoid sarcasm and put downs when you disagree? Those are all signs that you have a balanced relationship, and that you'll bring that sense of give-and-take to your sexual relationship, too.

Do you know the names of their brothers and sisters? Parents? Best friends?

Who we are has a lot to do with the people around us. Even if you haven't met them yet, it's a good sign if you and your partner have at least talked about the other people who are important in your lives. Does he hate his mom? Why? Was her dad never around? How does she feel about that? Who are his best friends and how did they become close?

Talking about your family and friends means that you talk about things that are important to both of you. It means that you share your feelings about the people who are closest to you, too. If you're not comfortable talking about these things, it probably means that you don't completely trust each other. And do you really think it's a good idea to have sex with someone you don't trust?

There's a saying that when you have sex with someone, you're really having sex with everyone they've ever had sex with. (Scary thought, right? That's why condoms are so

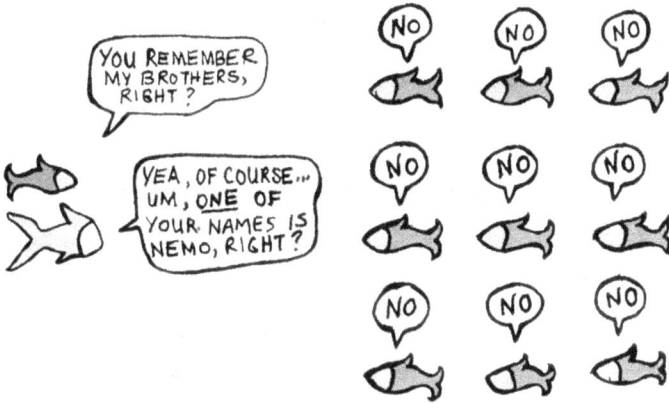

important.) When you get into a relationship with someone, in a way you're also getting into a relationship with everyone who is important to him or her—especially his or her family. Even if you've never met their family, your partner has been shaped more by their family experiences than by anything else in their life. What your partner knows about communicating, expressing feelings, resolving problems, and showing affection was learned in the context of family relationships. Knowing about your partner's family, and how he (or she) feels about it, is one of the best ways to get to know your partner.

Do you know what your partner's afraid of?

Fear and sex don't usually mix well. Some fears can be addressed pretty easily. For example, if you're worried about getting pregnant or catching an STD, the risks can be drastically reduced by taking a few simple precautions (like using a condom and another form of birth control every time you have sex). Other fears, like being emotionally or physically hurt, or fearing the consequences of going against your own morals or your family's expectations, are more complex.

Everyone's afraid of something, whether it's something as big as abandonment or as small as a spider. If you know what your partner's afraid of, you'll have an easier time talking about it when one of you is feeling scared or vulnerable, rather than having it blow up or get buried. Those things usually just add to the hurt or fear.

And if your partner's afraid of having sex, even though he

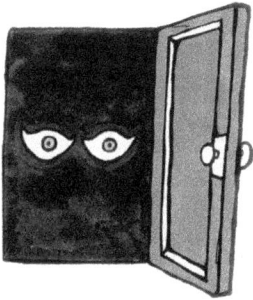

or she may want to, that's something you need to know too. Maybe he's had a previous bad experience. She may be concealing something that happened to her in the past because she's embarrassed or ashamed or because it's painful for her to think about, much less talk about.

Having sex can strengthen a relationship, but it can also destroy it if it doesn't feel right. And the only way to way to make sure it feels right is if both of you are comfortable and informed. So ask your partner what she (or he) is afraid of. Share your own fears and concerns. If you're close enough to be having sex, you should be close enough to discuss your fears.

Have you asked your partner, "Is there anything I should know about you before we have sex?"

"Why didn't you tell me?"

"You didn't ask."

Sound familiar?

When it comes to sex, what you don't know *can* hurt you—like if your partner has a sexually transmitted disease, for example. They may not have kept the information from you because they wanted to hurt you; they might just have been too embarrassed or ashamed or afraid of how you would react. By asking the question at the top of this page, you open the door for someone to tell you something she (or he) may have wanted to say but was too shy to bring up on her (or his) own.

You have to be serious when you ask this question, even if

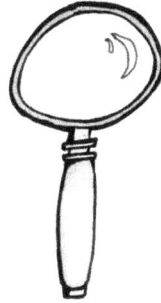

the other person looks at you uncom-
fortably or laughs. Asking the question shows that you have at least one
important qualification for having a sexual
relationship—sensitivity to your partner and
openness to hearing his or her concerns.

You also may be surprised at the answers you get to this
question. Here are just a few things that your partner might
say: "It's my first time," "I'm married," "My mom will kill
me if she finds out," "I'm pregnant," "I have herpes," "I'm
HIV positive," "I'm having my period," "I was abused by my
stepfather and I don't know how I feel about doing this," "I
prefer to do it outside, under the stars," "I love you."

Ask. You'll be glad you did.

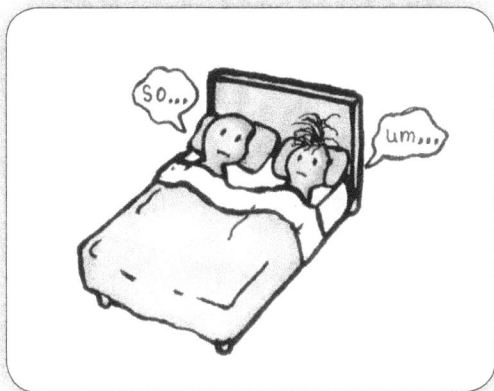

Getting to Know Your Partner
Teens Share Their Experiences

Rush to Love

By Jennifer Ramos

Growing up, I felt like I needed to have love. I'd watch romantic movies and TV shows and think, "Why don't I have what they have?" I felt like love could change everything. I thought that when I got older, I'd be able to experience that. But it didn't exactly happen that way. Instead of suddenly meeting a guy, connecting, and falling in love, I went through guy after guy after guy.

When I was younger, guys didn't notice me. But when I was 14, I started getting a lot of male attention. I found that extremely flattering, and I wanted to go out with them before the attraction went away.

Every time a guy came up to me, I imagined it would be like the movies. I thought it would only take one try to find love. In 8th grade, I met my first boyfriend, Eddy. He wrote me a letter in class telling me how much he liked me, how cute he thought I was, and how much he'd like to go out with me.

When I got the note, I was surprised. I'd noticed him before and thought he was really cute, with green eyes, dirty blond hair, and a baby face. But I knew absolutely nothing about him.

The only thing I felt I needed to know was that he had an interest in me. I didn't think I needed to find out much more to fall in love, because that's not how it happened in the movies I saw.

After that, we were officially boyfriend and girlfriend. We never discussed our relationship, but whenever anyone asked if we went out, we'd say yes. We talked, we kissed, we held hands. I was excited about having a boyfriend, but at the same time I was disappointed.

I saw how people in the movies acted: strange, in a good way, never wanting to be away from each other. They'd get lost in their loved one's eyes. But when I was with Eddy, I felt nothing. He seemed more into his friends and being cool than he was into being with me. The connection wasn't there. We broke up after a month and a half.

About a week or two later, I started going out with his friend Nelson. I liked being with Nelson because he was funny. Then I went out with Ryan, who was athletic. After Ryan, there was Alan. He was a thrill to be with because he was wild and would do anything, without any worries.

I went out with each of them for about two months. Either I didn't like them enough to stay with them or they cheated on me. I was usually the one to call it off. I was too eager to find my true love. I dove into each new relationship without really knowing anything about the person I was with.

Then it hit me — love. It was a beautiful September day. I was walking through a park with my friend Diana, when we ran into Dan, who Diana knew from school. He pulled her to the side and asked her questions about me, then we all sat in the park and talked for a while.

Dan was tall, thin and muscular, with a wonderful smile and gorgeous eyes. He seemed nice and I was attracted to him. I gave him my number so that we could talk some more.

After we talked a few times about our lives and interests, we became a couple. We went out to the park for walks. Our walks felt so calm, so different from my other relationships. I felt like I could connect with Dan.

Dan was sweet, asking questions about my day and showing concern about my feelings by asking about any little emotion I expressed. He'd bug out with me sometimes, like when I wanted to watch cartoons or play kid games.

Dan told me that he was in a gang, but I didn't mind because I thought that love would save him. By October, I was beginning to have very strong feelings for him. I felt like I could love him. I finally felt like the people in the movies.

By November, we were having sex. I'd had sex once before with Alan, which was a mistake. When I lost my virginity, it was to get it over with, but when I was with Dan, it was more sensual and emotional. I experimented sexually with him instead of just having sex. I felt closer to Dan after we did it. I felt so comfortable and free with him. I felt like this was it.

On Christmas, he took me ice skating. The sky was clear and the moon shone down on us while we skated around the rink. It was so romantic. Then, as we skated around, he proposed to me. It was just like a scene from a movie. The scenery was perfect and the moment was right. I believed I was in love with him so much, so I said, "Yes."

I was so excited that this was happening to me. I finally found the guy I was going to spend the rest of my life with. Emotionally and physically, I felt like we were already married. I even designed a tattoo for us to get, a made-up symbol that represented our love.

Every time a guy came up to me, I imagined it would be like the movies.

But by March, the things that I thought love would fix, like his being in a gang, became hard to deal with. He hadn't talked about the gang much before he proposed, because he knew I didn't like it. But now he started making references to his gang and his status in most of our conversations. He and a few of his friends also chased Chinese delivery guys and stole their food for fun. I guess he thought I'd be all right with it, but I wasn't.

I had thought our love would overpower the bad things, but I was wrong. Our relationship started to go downhill. We didn't go places anymore. All we did was go to his house to fool around. It wasn't at all like the movies now.

I didn't want him to be my boyfriend anymore, but I wasn't sure I wanted to go through breaking up with him, either. I didn't want to be in search of love again. I told myself I could deal with not having the "perfect man" as long as I still had the company.

But I talked to my best friend about how unhappy I was. He asked me questions that made me think about how I was feeling. In June, I broke up with Dan. His facial expression was blank. I don't know if he was hurt or relieved.

After our relationship ended, I felt like he'd been there just to fulfill my need to be in love. I might have fooled myself into believing that I was in love with him because he was the first guy who treated me decently. I wish I hadn't let Dan into my life so quickly. I think if I'd known him better, I'd never have fallen in love with him.

I had thought our love would overpower the bad things, but I was wrong.

Even though I was relieved to be away from him, I still missed him. Breaking up with someone I thought I'd spend my life with made me think hard about relationships. I realized that all of my relationships were rushed; we'd meet and become boyfriend and girlfriend right away.

I realized I should get to know the person I'm attracted to before I decide to play with my emotions. I learned that it's not healthy for me to have such a big need for love, because it just leads me to jump into relationships. Then it hurts too much when I end up not having the love I'm looking for.

I haven't had a boyfriend since I broke up with Dan, and that's fine. I've been dating, though. Dating for me is going places, talking, and getting to know someone—and that's it. It's not being a couple.

I feel like I'm in control now because I can speak to or date a guy without having that question stuck in my mind: "Is he my soul mate?" I don't feel the need to try on a relationship just to find out. I'm more likely to find that out if I get to know the person first.

Dating is fun, now that I don't jump into things. Love is something I can wait for.

Jennifer was 17 when she wrote this story.

Opening Up to My Girl

By Antwaun Garcia

Once in a while someone finally grows up and realizes what he wants. In my case, I went from being what you would call a pimp, a playa, someone who doesn't care about other people's feelings, to someone who is trying hard to settle down and be caring.

In all of my previous relationships I have cheated on a female with one or numerous other females. I didn't care too much about their feelings. I used females like a boy uses a toy.

Back in those days I used to have what I called "a phase" with a female. I would gas her head up like I needed her, like she was everything to me. (It was easy for me to tell girls nice things when I didn't mean them.) Then, poof, out of nowhere I'd let her know it was over. I could never face rejection so I would hand it out before it came to me.

I could never face rejection so I would hand it out before it came to me.

I would toss her number away, toss her letters, toss any pics of us, too. Kind of cold-hearted, I know, but it's the truth.

I would have females depressed thinking about me, wondering what I might be doing. My way of getting over a female was to just bag another one. Then, once again, after about a month, it was "bye-bye."

I knew I didn't want to be like two of my boys, who were almost devastated because their girls left them. I'd hear cats in the streets complaining, "My girl left me." But that wasn't my way.

But after a while, I started getting annoyed at females who only cared how thick my pockets were. I wanted to settle down, to have a girl to go places with and to miss when she wasn't with me.

Now, believe it or not, I think I have found that one. At the time we started talking, I was talking to five other girls, and she was talking to some cornball around her way. We were both tired of these corny people and wanted something serious. I will admit, I wasn't planning to be faithful to her at first. But she opened my eyes to the fact that she wasn't a dummy I could talk to and get my way with.

Now I have been dating her for the past 10 months, and they have been the best 10 months I have ever spent with any girl. She is mad cool and mad funny. She has a great personality and is a very good listener. Normally I don't talk to anyone, but my shorty has always opened her ear to me.

One week, we were talking on the phone from 10 at night to 4 in the morning when we both had to be at school early the next day. It wasn't one of those boring convos like, "The sky is blue, and the grass is green." We were really talking, really getting to know one another, really laughing the whole six or seven hours on the phone each day of that week. I had never done that with any female before.

I couldn't get enough of this girl. When we had class together we would sit next to one another and talk through the whole class, or write notes and crack jokes. Afterwards we would get something to eat up the block at the bagel shop, and then I would walk her to the bus. We did that from February to the end of the school year.

What's real interesting is we have nothing in common yet we are so compatible. She loves bacon. I hate pork. She loves horror films. I think they are corny and prefer a comedy or action film. She listens to rock and roll, and I listen to r&b and rap. Yet we still find similarities within one another.

And over the last 10 months, she has always been there for me, no matter what. I have been through some tough times, and she stood by me through it all. She listened when I talked about my life and past. She couldn't believe how I survived what I've been through. It kind of left her speechless. But telling her about my past helped her understand why I am the person I am. She loves me for who I am.

The main problem I have with her and most females I've liked is letting my feelings show. Don't get me wrong, I've told females what they want to hear, but usually when I don't mean it. It's hard for me to tell my feelings when they're real. After all, I have kept my feelings bottled up since I was 10, the year two of my best friends died. They were the only two people I confided my feelings to. When I lost them, I felt like I couldn't talk to anyone else, and not talking about my feelings became a habit.

> **I decided that growing in relationships is all about showing people how you feel, and taking a chance by trusting them with your soft side.**

But with my shorty, I wanted to tell her my feelings. It just seemed like a big risk. What if I told her how I felt and then we ended things? Then I might feel mad and stupid for showing her my vulnerable side. I might be heartbroken, or feel pitiful and depressed.

But I knew I'd feel just as bad if the relationship ended and I never told her how I felt, or, worse, if it ended *because* I never told her how I felt. I decided that growing in relationships is all about showing people how you feel, and taking a chance by trusting them with your soft side.

Even if there are grimy people in the world, that didn't mean my shorty was one of them, and that I couldn't work at letting my feelings show, at my own pace. And I wanted to get better at showing my feelings not just for my shorty, but because I wanted to be able to show my feelings to my family, too.

First I started by trying to tell her all I thought and felt, the good as well as the bad. Then I started trying to express the emotions I would rather not expose, like telling her when I missed her. She responds like any typical female. She says stuff like, "That was so cute."

But even though I'm getting more comfortable telling her what I think and feel, expressing those emotions I don't feel like talking about isn't getting easier. Sometimes my girlfriend won't realize how hard it is for me, and she will change the subject or even start singing or acting stupid when I'm about to say something I really need to say. That's when I think, "Either I'm boring her or she don't want to hear it." Then I stop talking and don't say anything more until she asks me to. It takes a lot of trust to expose my innermost thoughts and feelings. It can be frightening to trust her because if she breaks my trust I will feel worse.

Now that we are getting deeper into the relationship, my feelings are growing. We talk every night. No matter the time, we always make sure we put one another to sleep. But at the same time, I am still taking my time with showing her my feelings, because we both don't want to rush into something we are not ready for.

As I am growing older and more mature, I don't find the same things fun anymore. The idea of playing a female intentionally just doesn't sound fun. What sounds better is trying to build a good relationship by working to trust and be trustworthy, and showing my feelings more. I am respecting females a little more, and I'm feeling the benefits of it.

Antwaun was 18 when he wrote this story. He later attended college and became a manager at Home Depot.

Trusting Him With the Truth

By Anne Ueland

When I first started my job working at a daycare center, I met a handsome-looking boy named Cliff Jean-Michael. He was at the center to drop off his little sister. I couldn't keep my eyes off him. He looked so friendly and sweet.

When he came over to tell me his name, I couldn't help noticing his uniform, and that he was getting ready to go to work at a sneaker store. It was near the daycare center, so when I took my lunch break, I stopped by.

When I went inside, the first person I saw was Cliff. I put on a big smile and asked him if his store had a new style I was looking for. I didn't even think he remembered me from that morning.

I really liked him a lot. I even had this weird thought in my head to ask his sister if he had a girlfriend. I didn't, but I did look at his sister's last name and imagine how it would go with my first name. Anne Jean-Michael.

Then it happened. I was about to leave work for the day when Cliff came to the daycare. He told me he was not going to pick up his sister yet. He wanted to get a haircut and did I want to come with him? Of course I was loving the idea. It would give us the chance to know each other more.

On our way, Cliff asked me a lot of questions. One of them was about where I lived. I live in the foster care system, in a group home, but I lied to him. I told him that I lived with my mother. In the back of my mind I was thinking, "Why am I lying to this boy?"

I think I was afraid that if he knew the truth he might judge me and not want to get to know me. After all, some people put down girls in group homes. People say they are fast with boys, slow in school, and that no wants them.

When we got to the barber shop, I sat in a chair while Cliff got his hair cut. I couldn't help looking at him in the mirror. I saw him look at me, too.

When he was done he walked me to the subway and asked if I had a boyfriend. I said, "No," and I asked if he had a girlfriend. He said, "No," too.

At the station, I was about to go through the turnstile when Cliff said, "Wait. Let me ask you a question."

I said, "Go ahead."

"I was wondering if you wanted to go out with me."

"Yes," I said, and asked Cliff to come downstairs and wait for my train with me so we could talk. When my train came I gave Cliff a big hug and said, "I'll see you tomorrow."

After I started dating Cliff, I loved getting up early in the morning even though I am not a morning person. I knew I was getting up to see my boo.

I was afraid that if he knew I was in foster care he might judge me and not want to get to know me.

Cliff seemed to have a lot of good values. He did not smoke or drink. He went to school and got good grades. He even went to church on Sundays. I like a guy who has good values in life. I do not like guys that seem like they're going down the wrong road.

For some strange reason, Cliff made me feel whole inside. He always knew how to keep a smile on my face.

One day when I got off work, Cliff and I went to Central Park. We sat on some rocks and we started talking about how long we thought our relationship was going to last. I looked him in the eyes and said, "I think

I am falling in love with you." He said that he felt the same way, and we started to kiss.

I remember getting home and smiling and listening to love songs all night long. Even the staff at my group home, Ms. Trusty, asked me if I was in love.

Cliff would call me every day, sometimes more than twice a day. Cliff would talk about any issues that he had with his family. I also shared personal things about myself with him, but I still didn't talk about the fact that I was in a group home and the problems that went on there. I wanted to talk to him about these things, but I was still worried about what he'd think of me. When Cliff called me he would always ask, "Who was that lady who answered the phone?" I would say, "My mother," when it was really my staff.

Before school started, Cliff invited me to come to church to meet his family. When I met them, his family seemed very nice and friendly. During the service, Cliff kept smiling at his friends, which made me think that he was really happy to be with me. After the service he brought me upstairs where people were serving cakes and drinks. Cliff told his friends that I was his girlfriend. The way he said it made me feel good. I knew he was not ashamed of me.

The more I knew Cliff the more I wanted him to know all about me, too. Cliff always told me that I could share my deepest and darkest secrets with him and he would not think of me any differently. And I believed him, but for some reason I still could not tell him the truth. I felt bad inside that I was lying to him, because he seemed to care a lot about me. He had become a big support in my life. But I kept lying.

After a while the lies were really getting to me. Sometimes I couldn't even remember what lie I told him to cover up the fact that I lived in the group home. And when I had problems in the group home, I couldn't tell him why I was upset. I'd either have to pretend not to be upset or make up some other lie about why I was. Sometimes I would be moody toward him or take out my anger on him. Every time he would ask me what was wrong, I would tell him, "Nothing."

Everyone in my house told me that in order to have an open relation-ship I had to tell Cliff the truth about where I lived. But I was thinking to myself that it was too late. I had already lied to him. If I told him the truth now, I might lose him.

We'd known each other almost a year the spring that I finally told Cliff I lived in a group home. I remember the day well. I was walking him to his job and I told him. I'd gotten so tired of lying to him, plus I wanted him to know why I was so stressed out a lot of the time.

To my surprise, Cliff wasn't surprised. He said that he already knew. He said that one day he called my house and a person answered the phone and said, "107." He asked her what it stood for and she said, "This is a group home." He didn't say anything to me about it because he wanted to know how long it would be until I told him the truth.

Now I feel I can tell Cliff more about me and all I've gone through.

When I explained the reasons why I hadn't told him, Cliff understood. Since then, we've become even closer. Now I feel I can tell him more about me and all I've gone through.

That summer Cliff took me to a lot of differ-ent events with his church. I will never forget the day that we went to an amusement park. While we were at the park, it started raining hard, but we went on all the rides and had so much fun. It felt so good to be with him even though it was raining outside. On the bus back, we fell asleep on each other. I thought that was real special. To be wrapped up in his arms.

Then there was the time Cliff invited me to go to field day with his church. I was upset that day because everyone there was with family. I felt so bad that I was without family that I even started crying. Cliff asked me what was wrong and I told him that I wished my mother would change because I miss her.

Cliff gave me a hug and said, "Everything is going to be all right." He comforted me the whole way back. That's what I call a good boyfriend.

Cliff has helped me grow over the past year and seven months that we have been together. I have grown to be open with Cliff and express what I feel. I also learned that there is nothing wrong with being in a group home. I am not afraid to tell anyone that I live in one anymore. I think that people have no right to judge us, the kids who live in them. We are still all humans. Cliff has helped show me this by letting me be me.

Anne was 15 when she wrote this story.

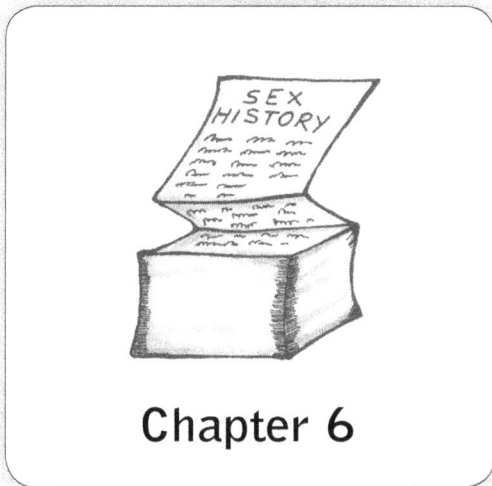

Chapter 6

Five Things to Ask Your Partner About Sex

Do you know how your partner learned about sex? Do you know what she or he learned?

What were the earliest messages your partner got about sex? Did she learn that sex was wonderful (but only after marriage)? Did he learn it was dirty and best kept secret? Did she learn it was a way to catch a man? Did he learn it was a way to prove his manliness?

SEX = *Dirty*

Why is it important to know about this stuff? Let's say, for example, that you learned that sex is the way to *keep a man*, but the man you're with learned that having sex with a lot of different people is the best way to *feel like a man*. One of you (or both of you) is going to be very disappointed with your relationship.

Or maybe your partner's knowledge of sex is based completely on watching Internet porn. He or she may have

SEX = *Love* some unrealistic or even harmful ideas of what sex is supposed to be like—including the idea that sex should be degrading or humiliating to one or both partners.

Because it's very common for people to have different ideas about sex depending on how they were raised, their experiences, or their religious beliefs, it's important for you and your partner to do some talking before you go there. Understanding what the other person wants and expects from a sexual relationship increases the chances that you will both feel comfortable and satisfied when you do start having sex.

SEX = ?

Do you know if your partner has been tested for STDs?

It's not easy to ask questions like: "Have you ever had unprotected sex?" and "Have you been tested for or had an STD?" Having this conversation will probably make you feel pretty awkward. But if you're too embarrassed to ask about STDs, you might end up with one, possibly HIV.

Before you have sex with someone, know what kind of risk you're taking. Just say it straight out: "We need to talk about a few things, like, I need to know if you've had sex before and if you've been tested for HIV and other STDs." (And beware: even if you ask the question, that doesn't mean you're going to get an honest answer. Many people

who have STDs *don't know* they have them.
It's also not uncommon for people to lie
about this kind of thing. That's why you
should always practice protected sex,
even if your partner says that he or she
has never had an STD.)

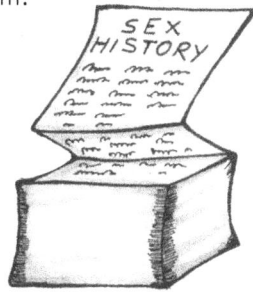

You may also want to ask your partner
to get tested. Tell them: "I'm going to do the same for you."
It may feel like you're putting your partner on the spot, but
it'll get easier.

Have you talked about what kind of contraception you'll use?

Having sex is a shared experience, and figuring out what kind of contraception you'll use should be a shared responsibility.

If you just assume that he's going to buy the condoms, or that she's on the pill, you might be in for an unpleasant surprise. You don't want to be in the heat of passion and find out that neither of you has protection.

If your partner's not being responsible about protection and you're planning to have sex anyway, then you need to go on birth control, or bring the condoms, or (ideally) both. But it's better for the two of you to talk about what kind of protection you're going to use, who's going to get it, and who's going to pay for it. Just talking about your feelings and plans for birth control and disease prevention is a good way to get to know each other better and feel more comfortable with each other. Sharing the responsibility for making sex safer can help you build trust.

And if your partner's pressuring you to have sex without birth control and a condom, start thinking about putting the sex plans on hold.

Have you talked about what you would do if you got pregnant (or got her pregnant)?

Many teenagers don't want to think about the possibility of getting pregnant, much less talk about it. But it's better to discuss what you would do if it happens—before it happens. Pregnancy is stressful enough without finding out at the last minute that you and your partner completely disagree about whether to have an abortion or have a baby. If you and your partner disagree about what to do, it will be even harder to figure out how to cope.

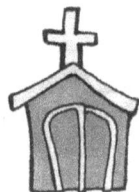

If the girl wants to have an abortion, and the guy doesn't agree, he might end up pressuring her to make a decision that she will regret later. If the girl wants to have and keep the baby, and the guy doesn't, the odds are that she'll end up raising the child alone. Meanwhile, he'll be legally responsible for paying child sup-

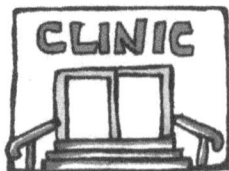

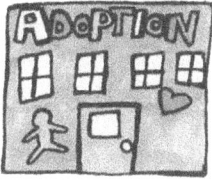

port even though he doesn't want to be a father.

If one or both of you think having a baby together might be exciting or bring you closer, remember that having a baby and raising a baby are two different things. Just because a guy says "I want you to have my baby," doesn't mean he's committing to sticking around for 18 years to raise it.

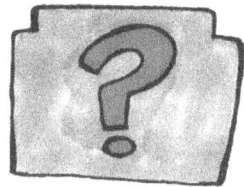

If you're not ready to raise a child at this point in your life, make sure your partner knows that—and do everything you can to keep it from happening. That means using birth control every single time you have sex, or not having sex till you're ready to have kids.

Will you be able to ask for what you want?

Being attracted to someone, even being in love, doesn't guarantee that you're going to have great sex. (Although it's a really good place to start!) In addition to being attracted and/or in love, you and your partner have to learn to touch each other in the right places, at the right times, in the right ways. By right we mean what's right for you. When it comes to sex, everyone has different turn-ons and turn-offs.

You shouldn't assume that your partner is just going to know instinctively what will excite you. There will be times when you find yourself thinking, "Faster" or "Slower" or "Over to the left." But will you be able to say it out loud? Will you be comfortable enough with your partner and with your own body to ask

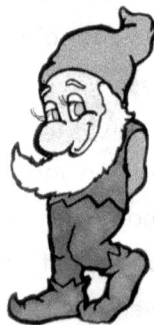

to be caressed or licked in just the right spot? Or to say, "That hurts," or "I don't like the way that feels"? Being able to overcome shyness and embarrassment in order to express your own desires and ask your partner to share his (or hers) is one sign that you might be mature enough to handle sex.

And when something doesn't feel right to you or you're just not ready, you should also always be able to say, "I don't want to." Someone who cares about you will not get angry, or act hurt, or try to make you feel guilty because you don't want to do something that makes you uncomfortable.

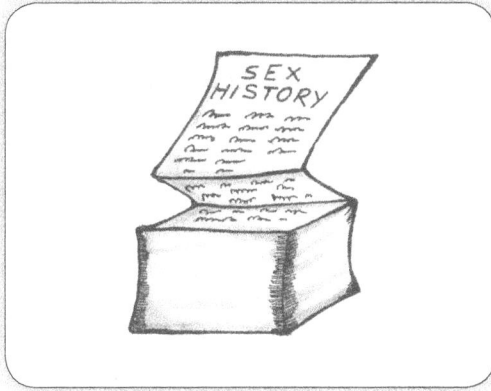

Having Better Sex
Teens Share Their Experiences

Performance Anxiety

By Anonymous

I'm 18, and have been sexually active for a little more than a year now. Having sex was a big step that, sadly, I don't think I was ready for. I once believed you should only have sex with someone you love. And, at the time I was with her, I felt I loved Beth, the first person I had sex with.

I enjoyed being with her physically in the beginning of our relationship, before we started having sex. But Beth wanted more. She was a virgin too. When we kissed, she took it further and further. I was no angel either, mind you, but she usually took the initiative and started to pressure me into having sex.

"But we can't have sex. I don't have a condom," was my usual excuse. Even though my hormones were raging, I had stage fright. I wanted our first time to be magic. I wanted to be a thrilling performer, and wasn't sure how she'd rate me.

One night, three months into our relationship, we were lying down in my room.

"Let's just do it already. I want to see what everybody is talking about," Beth whispered.

"Maybe next time, if we have a condom," I said.

Then she reached over the side of the bed, went through her bag, and pulled out a condom. She handed it to me. "Put it on, then," she said.

I was stunned. I couldn't think of any more excuses or anything else to say. And I felt overcome with lust. So I put it on and we had sex. I barely remember what it felt like, but it sure as hell didn't seem special.

I didn't openly talk about how I felt about the sex because I didn't want to risk hurting her feelings. I hoped that the more we had sex, the better it would become.

But the more sex we had, the less I felt for her. I was upset with myself for continuing to sleep with her but didn't have the heart to say, "I don't want to have sex with you anymore."

So my issues got expressed in other ways. I couldn't ejaculate, which added stress to the relationship. I could make her have an orgasm, and was happy about that, but she felt guilty about not being able to return the favor. "There's no reason to feel guilty," I told Beth one night. "It's not your fault."

I barely remember what my first time felt like, but it sure as hell didn't seem special.

"But if I can't make you orgasm, why should I let you do it to me all the time?" she asked.

Even though I tried to reassure her and not dwell on my problem, I did feel left out. I was jealous of her because I wasn't able to have an orgasm. And I didn't understand why. I was embarrassed by my problem, and had a hard time talking about it with anyone.

I never raised the issue with Beth, and she only mentioned it in the form of little jokes. I felt that her humor was mean-spirited because even after I told her that her jokes bothered me, she didn't stop. I tried to talk to my parents about it and they were each like, "I don't want to know." They knew I had sex, but didn't want to know the details. I was very frustrated.

Beth and I broke up after eight months. But my problem persisted with other girls I slept with. After a while, my main satisfaction during sex was making the other person have an orgasm.

I started to think that I needed to talk to a doctor. I was concerned that something was physically wrong with me. In May, I made an appointment at a teen center that has a free clinic. Once there, I received a general checkup and got tested for STDs by my doctor. Doc sure did love to talk, asking me about my sex life, what I'm interested in, and what I want to do when I get older. His talking made me feel more comfortable.

But I still felt very awkward confiding in this older gentleman about my ejaculation issues, particularly after he'd inserted a small cotton swab into the urethra of my penis for examination purposes.

Three weeks later, I went back for my results. Doc told me that my tests came back negative and that I didn't have anything physically wrong with me to prevent me from ejaculating. So he gave me some advice on how to solve my problem.

He said that maybe I just didn't feel comfortable having sex yet and the anxiety was preventing me from climaxing. He also said that, if I continued to have sex, I needed to relax more and not obsess about my performance.

He suggested that I masturbate with my partner and have her participate more with my masturbation during each session. We could then move on to oral sex and gradually begin having intercourse until, finally, I felt comfortable having sex without the masturbation.

I followed his suggestions over the summer and found that, by the end of August, I was able to have an orgasm with my partner. Sometimes I'm still not able to come, but my problem doesn't bother me as much as it used to. I'm so thankful to Doc and the clinic.

Still, even though I'm enjoying sex more, I think I should've waited. And I definitely shouldn't have had sex with Beth. Succumbing to pressure in silence just led to months of frustration and embarrassment. And it didn't allow me to experience my first few times as something special.

The author was in high school when he wrote this story.

Love Made Me Carefree... and Careless

By Lenny Jones

Last year I decided to ring in the New Year with a bang. I spent New Year's Eve in New York with my girlfriend, Infatuation (not her real name, of course). I took her out to a popular Broadway show. Afterward, we planned to watch the ball drop at Times Square and have dinner at my place.

I had liked Infatuation since the first time I laid eyes on her. She was pretty and funny, but I thought she was beyond my league. She liked the older, taller, pretty-boy types who did the GQ dress code. For a whole year I tried and tried to go out with her, but she'd reject me time and time again.

Then we lost contact for almost a year. The day I saw her again, all my feelings for her resurfaced big time. My eyes glowed and I felt this rush of giddiness. When I ended up kissing her that same day I thought I was on top of the world.

We finally did go out, and I did everything I could for her—took her for long walks in the park, talked on the phone for hours, took her to the movies, partying and clubbing, anything she wanted. I wanted to be the best guy she'd ever been with.

So you can imagine how I felt spending New Year's Eve with Infatuation. I wanted it to blow her away and make it truly be a night to remember—and it was, but for the wrong reason.

We were going to stay out until the ball dropped, but it was freezing, so we went back to my place to warm up. We ordered Chinese and watched the ball drop on TV.

Later, in bed, I lay beside her and started tickling her. We started kissing and caressing each other. We were having a great time. We undressed each other in the dark. After a while, it was time to do the deed. I was so excited—we'd never had sex before.

I had always wondered how sex would be without protection. I was dying to find out. I really liked Infatuation—hell, I loved this girl and thought she was the perfect person for me. I didn't want to have sex with her...I wanted to make love. I thought that this was the chance of a lifetime to show her my stuff.

I started thinking to myself, "Should I put on a condom?" I didn't want anything to spoil this moment. What if she lost the mood and couldn't get it back? Besides, I felt it would be degrading her if I did. I didn't want to make her think I thought she was dirty.

> **I didn't want anything to spoil this moment. What if she lost the mood and couldn't get it back?**

Half of me was telling me to put one on, but the other half was on a roll, telling me to indulge myself. Even the thought of getting her pregnant didn't scare me. For some sick reason, I thought if I did get her pregnant, that would just make our future together more secure.

It wasn't like I didn't have any condoms around. I had some right under my bed, but I didn't bother to reach for them. I figured it was a new year, why not get a little freaky?

But then I thought, "It wouldn't be right to make a decision like that without her consent," so I asked her, "Should I put on a condom?" She just turned her head and moaned. It wasn't a yes or no, it was more like a "Let's do it already, what are you waiting for?"

So I took one last look at myself and said, "Oh, what the hell," and we did it...no condom, nothing.

I have to admit that it did feel good at the time—a little too good. Soon I came to a startling conclusion...I was bone dry! I had always worn condoms before and could tell when the end was near, but this time I was caught by surprise.

I started to freak out. I kept saying to myself, "I hope I didn't come inside her," and, "Oh my God, what have I done?"

I didn't bother to tell her because I thought she knew. And if she didn't, I didn't want to mess up the night for her. She just went to sleep beside me, but I couldn't sleep. All I kept thinking was, "I might be a father."

The next day, when I got my nerve, I gave her a call and told her that I might have gotten her pregnant. She started crying and kept saying, "You're joking, right?" I felt really bad. I wanted to say I was joking but I wasn't. Then I told her not to worry, I would figure something out.

I started calling around to see if I could get her the "morning after pill" (also known as emergency contraception). Most of the places were closed for the holidays, and I didn't know then that you can get EC at a hospital. I found one clinic that was open, but they wanted to charge me $90 and I was flat broke.

The next day I made more calls but had no luck. I had one last hope and that was my brother. I asked him if I could borrow the $90, but he was broke, too. He said I should just wait and not worry about it. So I took his advice. I called Infatuation and she was OK about waiting to take a pregnancy test, too.

That night she came over again. It felt good being with her, talking to her face to face. The only problem was that she had some recurring stomach pains. She told me not to worry about them. But a few days later, her stomach started hurting her again. This time, the pain wouldn't go away. I ended up calling an ambulance.

We landed in the emergency room. The doctors examined Infatuation and ran tests. I asked what the diagnosis was, and they said she showed symptoms of PID—Pelvic Inflammatory Disease. Even though I had no idea what that was, I panicked.

I asked the doctor if it was sexually transmitted and she said, "Most likely." She also said I should get myself tested for gonorrhea and chlamydia.

Infatuation had to stay overnight. So I stayed right by her side and made two hard chairs into a makeshift bed. In the morning, the doctors wanted her to take an HIV test. When they said that, I felt butterflies in my stomach. All I could think was, "What did she give me?" But the test came out negative.

Infatuation and I didn't really talk too much during all this. I guess we were too scared. But I did reassure her that I would be there for her no matter what—and I meant it. She was my everything and I felt like I would have nothing without her. I barely even left her side. I waited on her hand and foot. But everything changed the next day.

Before all this happened, being with Infatuation had been like a natural high that made everything seem happier and shinier.

We were watching TV when all the doctors came in, and asked me to leave the room. As I left, I could feel my hands shaking. My elbows just went dead and my heart was racing. I was so scared. I paced up and down the hallways for at least an hour. In that time, I just talked myself out of being scared cause I had chosen not to be protected and the punishment would fit the crime.

When I went back to her room, Infatuation was sitting on the bed, crying. A rush of fear went through me but I told myself to take it like a man. She looked at me as though she wanted to kill me, her eyes all red and glassy. Then she asked me how many partners I had been with. It took me a little while to sort out the names and then I told her.

She started talking about how she had only been with one other guy, Plague (not his real name). Then I told her that she was the only girl I had done it with raw. With all the other girls I had been with, the condom was on 100% of the time.

She started defending Plague and we got into a really bad argument. She had never really told me much about Plague, but her blaming me made me realize she still had feelings for him and trusted him more than she trusted me. I asked her what she had that caused the PID and when I found out it was gonorrhea, I hunched forward into a ball. I almost cried.

Infatuation thought she'd spite me by calling up one of her friends and talking, in detail, about her sexual experiences with Plague. I tried to ignore it but couldn't. Then she called up one of her exes and started flirting with him right in front of my face. Tears started streaming down my cheeks and I couldn't take it anymore. I got up and headed toward the door.

She hung up the phone, jumped out of bed and grabbed my arm. She asked me not to leave and apologized, but by this time I was seeing red. I ended up cursing her out and telling her that I hated her and that my life would be better without her. I said so much stuff that I can hardly remember it all. Finally, she told me to leave.

After I took some time to cool off, I felt kind of messed up about all the things I said to hurt her. Even though I did feel betrayed, I shouldn't have said the things I did.

I started to consider the fact that she may have just been scared and angry. Maybe she didn't really mean to blame me. I started to sympathize with her and decided to apologize. But I knew deep down that I'd said too much. She wouldn't talk to me or anything.

A few days later, I called her up. I hoped that she had taken the time to rethink things. Before all this happened, being with Infatuation had been like a natural high that made everything seem happier and shinier. Without her, the brightness seemed to have disappeared. I still cared about her and I wanted us to work things out. She said she did, too.

I went back to the hospital the day she was getting discharged, thinking that we'd be love birds again. Her cousin was in her room when I got there, and Infatuation didn't really say anything to me. When we got outside, she walked off with her cousin as if I wasn't even there. When

I watched her walk away without a kiss, a hug or even a goodbye, I knew it was all over.

A few days later, I got myself checked out. I had tested positive for gonorrhea and chlamydia, so the doctor gave me some antibiotics. A few weeks later he gave me a clean bill of health. As for Infatuation, I never saw her again.

My experience with Infatuation was very traumatic. I had never cared about anyone as much as I cared for her, and look what happened. Now I'm afraid that if I ever feel as strongly for a girl as I did for Infatuation, I will put my health and well-being at risk again. I have this destructive, carefree attitude when I'm in love and can't seem to help it. But I hope I'm smarter next time, because after going through all that, I never want to have unprotected sex again.

I was lucky this time...I would have been screwed if she had HIV or something uncurable like herpes. I'm just happy I was able to walk away with everything intact. You may think I'm joking, but these days I won't even kiss a girl without a condom in my pocket.

Lenny was 21 when he wrote this story.

Put Yourself Before Sex

By Nicole Hawkins

Listening to most of my girl friends talk, it seems to me we are seriously confused about our place in this world. Time after time, I hear girls who have had sex say they didn't enjoy it. Yet in the same breath they rave about how good a guy is and how they wish he would call. They think having sex is more important than how they feel.

I wish I could teach girls what my father taught me: *You* come first. Pleasing a horny guy, if it means doing something that makes you feel bad, is a disservice to yourself.

It's not that I think sex is bad. I think good sex is good and bad sex is bad. But the worst thing is just to lie there as if you don't matter and hold your feelings inside. I hope I'm not coming off as someone who has got it 100% under control, 'cause I don't. But I do know from experience that if you're in a relationship with someone you trust, you can discuss just about everything under the sun.

I wish I could teach girls what my father taught me: *You* come first.

I have a good physical relationship with my boyfriend (which doesn't include intercourse). Everything is 50/50 and that's because anything I want to say, I say it. I don't regret anything I've done, probably because it was thoroughly thought through and not rushed.

I think a lot of girls my age and younger see sex as one of the few milestones of womanhood. First, you get your period. Then you get married and have sex, or vice versa. Finally you get pregnant. You're a wife, a mother, and a woman.

But I think you can be a woman without having sex. Sex doesn't define who you are. Being a woman means to me that you are independent, strong, intuitive, emotional, compassionate, intelligent, and unique.

When I'm a woman, I'll be able to walk up to people, shake their hands firmly and look them in the eye as I introduce myself. I'll live fully on my own and not depend on my dad for a few bucks here and there. I'll walk down the street in the sexiest and classiest outfit and not feel like an impostor. I'll be proud of being me.

I consider myself to be in the process of becoming a woman, and I know that having sex won't make it complete. Being true to myself and following my heart will. I hope that other girls can feel the same.

Nicole was 18 when she wrote this story.

How I Stopped Giving In

By Anonymous

Most of my experiences with sex have had very little to do with love and care. I've been dogged out by guys more times than I care to remember. Even my current boyfriend has often seemed more interested in getting his nut off than in talking with me or holding me meaningfully. Normally I go along with it just to make him happy. But in the last few months I've been learning that if I want to get respect, first I have to respect myself. I've started to speak up for what I want.

When I was 14, I knew this guy named Jamal with soft and curly dark brown hair, and a light-brown chocolate complexion. He was 19, but he acted so grown up—like he was 25. I wanted so badly for him to ask me to be his girl. I thought that going out with an older guy would make me look older, and then other older guys would notice me more.

One day Jamal and I were chilling in the attic of his house, drinking and smoking weed. We were sitting on a big soft couch in the dark watching television and he started to kiss me. The last thing I wanted to do was stop him; I thought he was starting to like me.

The next thing I knew, we were laying on the floor and Jamal said in a low voice, "I'm gonna put on a jimmy-hat, OK?" I just nodded my head and proceeded to take off my clothes. He went to the bathroom and stayed in there for what seemed like 15 minutes. "What's taking him so long?" I kept thinking.

When he finally came back, he still had his shirt on. "Let me see you," I asked suspiciously. I wanted to make sure that he really had on a condom. When he said no, in the back of my mind I was thinking, "Hold up, what's wrong with him?" but I was so drunk and high that I just went with the flow. It wasn't until about three weeks later, when I didn't get my period, that I found out Jamal hadn't had a condom on after all.

I was so scared that I kept my pregnancy hidden for about three and a half months. One time my sister was driving me to school, and I had morning sickness. Instead of telling her what was wrong, I just threw up in my mouth and swallowed the vomit back down.

My mother had a feeling that something was wrong with me, so she took me to her gynecologist. There, they found out for sure that I was pregnant and I decided to have an abortion.

Even after all that, I still wanted to be with Jamal (talk about being blind). The day after the abortion I went with my friend Natasha to his house. When we got there, he didn't even acknowledge the fact that we had sex together. "You know I was pregnant with your baby, right, Jamal?" I said to him.

"Oh, word?" he asked without seeming to care. "What happened?"

I told him about the abortion, hoping that he would show me a little compassion. "Oh" is all he said to me, like I was just one more girl that he had knocked up.

After Jamal, I got involved with a guy who used to punch me and curse at me. The only time that he was nice was when he wanted to have sex. I wouldn't leave him, though, because I didn't think I could do any better for myself.

After those and other experiences, it was hard for me to trust another guy. Then last April, I met Duane, my present boyfriend. The week after I started at my new school, he just walked up to me and started a conversation. We went to the McDonald's by our school, and the whole time I was thinking, "He's just trying to hit it."

Duane confessed to me that he and two other schoolmates had made a bet to see who could bag me first (I guess Duane won). Luckily for me he was being honest, because that told me to keep my eyes open and not to make myself vulnerable by falling in love with him.

After Duane told me about his little bet, it was even harder for me to believe that he wanted me for me. But I still gave him my number, and we started going out that day.

When we finally had sex, it was about a month into the relationship. I don't really enjoy sex that much. I was just doing it for Duane. We were in the basement of his house. I was so scared, because I didn't want Duane to tell all his boys in school that I let him hit the skins. "I hope you're for real," I remember telling him the whole time that we were having sex. "I don't want to get hurt again."

"I'm for real," he kept assuring me.

That first time Duane had asked me if I wanted to use a condom and I said yes. The next time we had sex, we didn't use one because neither of us had one. After that, if I brought it up he would try to manipulate me. One time he was kissing me seductively, and asked, "You want me to please you, right? If I can't feel you, how am I going to do that?"

> **I don't really enjoy sex that much. I was just doing it for Duane.**

I replied like I always did. "It's not about pleasing me," I said. "Because I don't get anything out of it anyway."

The kissing didn't do anything to me, really, because sex doesn't faze me. But, his groveling was a very pitiful sight. So, unfortunately, most of the time I just gave in.

The most annoying form of manipulation, though, was when he questioned my love for him. "If you loved me," he would tell me, "then you'd let me please you without a condom." Again, I would just give in.

I never really told Duane how I felt about unprotected sex or sex in general. The truth was, I hated the task of laying down knowing that I was going to do something that was tedious to me. Before I saw him I was always hoping he would just want to talk with me and find out what was on my mind. I would ask him for a condom before we had sex, but if he didn't have one we would do it anyway. That was that: No talk. No nothing. Just sex.

Lately, I've thought about the consequences that might result from unprotected sex, and I realize that taking care of my body is more important than making my man happy. I don't want anything more to happen as a result of my being irresponsible. I've already been pregnant twice. I'm not ready for a child now, and I worry that having another abortion could jeopardize the possibility of my having a family in the future.

But because I didn't communicate with Duane about how I felt he never took care of carrying a condom. On the other hand, neither did I. I always left it up to him. I thought it was his job even though I knew he didn't want to use one.

At the same time, the more Duane wanted to have sex without a condom, the more I believed that he just wanted me for my body. If I got pregnant, I figured he'd leave me.

I know, now, that if I don't want to have sex, then I don't have to.

One day after school, I went to his house like I usually did. Strangely, we were the only ones in the whole house that afternoon. As soon as he told me that we would have no interruption, I was disappointed. I knew what he had planned, and having sex was the last thing on my mind. I started watching television, to get him into something other than sex, but that didn't help any. He started kissing my neck, and I was getting angry. I pushed him away first, and when he wouldn't stop, I told him, "Stop, I'm watching TV."

"C'mon," Duane told me. "Let's just do this before everyone comes home." That, I think, is what sent me over the edge. I got so pissed at him. It seemed as if he wanted me to do a "quickie" for him so that he could get his nut off. That proved to me that the only thing he wanted from me was sex.

That's when I finally spoke up about how I felt. I told Duane straight up, "I really don't like having sex with you, or anyone for that matter. It doesn't do anything for me, 'cause it's not what I care about at this time in my life. I have to finish school first, and then do what I feel is right for me."

I let him know everything that was on my mind. I confided in him about how I just went along with the sex mainly to please him. I assured him, however, that I loved him and that his manhood had nothing to do with it. It was just a question of what I wanted for myself at that time. Even so, he still felt the need to defend himself. "What, I'm not good enough for you?" he kept saying. "I can't satisfy you?"

After that conversation, Duane tried harder to please me whenever we did have sex, and I started to feel hopeless about ever getting through to him. Every time he wanted to have sex and I didn't, either because he didn't have a condom or I just plain didn't want to, we would end up having sex anyway.

Duane thought that he had to satisfy me to keep me happy with him so I wouldn't have to look for pleasure somewhere else. If I said that I didn't want to have sex, and I was firm about it, then he would think that I was seeing someone else. He would also either pout or just go outside and not come back for the night.

He did that on two occasions. The second time I got so heated after he left me alone all night in his crib, worrying, that I screamed at him about the respect I deserve from him. After I gave Duane a piece of my mind, he realized that I wasn't joking around. Now he may be defiant once in a while, but overall, I've taken hold of our relationship.

Since I learned to communicate and to hold my ground, Duane now respects my wishes when I'm not in the mood. He also knows that if he doesn't have a condom then nothing sexual will happen between us. I've stopped giving in to his constant manipulating, and that has led him to stop trying to persuade me to do things I don't want to.

I know, now, that if I don't want to have sex, then I don't have to. I will only truly enjoy sex if I do it when I'm ready. If my man can't handle that and he wants to leave then it wasn't meant to be between us, and I still have time to find the right guy for me. It isn't worth it to have unsatisfying sex just to please your boyfriend. After a while, you start to dread doing it and can't make the sacrifice anymore.

Duane has grown up a lot, too. He understands that right now my education is the most important thing in my life and relationships are about walks in the park, long talks over the phone, communication (a biggie), and most importantly, love.

Personally, I think for sex to be enjoyable, both people have to be ready, know what they want and feel the same way about each other. They have to care deeply and use protection. That way, no one gets hurt.

I know now that I wasn't ready for sex, and I don't know that I ever will be. First, I need to get my priorities straight. My plan is to finish high school, start college, learn to depend on myself by living alone, getting a job, and living life to the fullest. But if I do things that I am not ready for now then I won't be able to achieve these goals.

The author was in high school when she wrote this story.

How to Handle the Reluctant Condom Wearer

If your partner says: I don't like using condoms.
You can say: Why not?

If your partner says: It doesn't feel as good with a condom.
You can say: I'll feel more relaxed. If I'm more relaxed, I can make it feel better for you.

If your partner says: But we've never used a condom before.
You can say: I don't want to take any more risks.

If your partner says: Condoms are gross.
You can say: Being pregnant when I don't want to be is worse. So is getting AIDS.

If your partner says: Don't you trust me?
You can say: Trust isn't the point. People carry infections without knowing it. And trust won't keep me from getting pregnant.

If your partner says: I'll pull out.
You can say: That's still risky. Pre-cum can carry infections, and I could still get pregnant.

If your partner says: Condoms aren't romantic.
You can say: Worrying about pregnancy and STDs is even less romantic.

If your partner says: Making love with a condom on is like taking a shower with a raincoat on.
You can say: Well, doing it without a condom is playing with my life.

If your partner says: It just isn't as sensitive.
You can say: With a condom, you might last even longer, and that'll make up for it.

If your partner says: I don't stay hard when I put on a condom.
You can say: I can do something about that.

If your partner says: Putting it on spoils the mood.
You can say: Not if I help put it on.

If your partner says: I'll try, but it might not work.
You can say: Practice makes perfect.

If your partner says: But I love you.
You can say: Then you'll help me protect myself.

If your partner says: I guess you don't really love me.
You can say: I'm not going to "prove my love" by risking my life.

If your partner says: Just this once without it. Just the first time.
You can say: It only takes once to get pregnant. It only takes once to get an infection. It only takes once to get AIDS.

If your partner says: I'm not using one, no matter what.
You can say: Well, then I guess we're not having sex.

Adapted from Planned Parenthood (www.plannedparenthood.org).

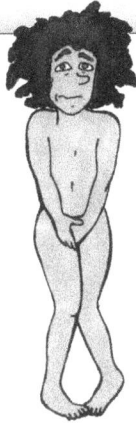

Chapter 7

Five Things to Ask About Each Other's Bodies

Do you *really* like to kiss him (or her)?

Kissing is part of sex—and for most people it's a really fun part. Kissing is how you get warmed up. Some kisses show how sweet you can be; others show your passion. Your responsiveness when being kissed and kissing back makes your partner feel desirable and cared for.

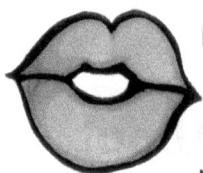

Kissing is how you begin to get to know someone sexually. It's one way you learn what the other person likes in a physical relationship—and what makes her uncomfortable. It's a way to show what turns you on. It gives both of you a chance to express your feelings and get to know each other better. And it can be really fun and exciting even if it doesn't lead to anything else.

Kissing is a way to get some of the pleasure that comes from sex without danger or serious consequences. Kissing creates a bond and helps make you feel safe with your partner. If your partner wants to stop kissing, and you get the message and stop, it tells them that you're trustworthy and considerate.

Do you know what they look like without their hair combed or their makeup on (and do they know what you look like)?

Sex is messy. You don't keep your composure. You might fall asleep afterwards (and drool on the pillow). So if you're afraid of what you or your partner are going to look like the next morning—if you feel like you don't want your partner to see what you look like after sweating and messing up your hair—then wait. Work up to it. Go on a date without any makeup and see how he reacts. Get caught in the rain. Go out in public together on a bad hair day (and don't wear a hat!). Stay together one night but don't have sex and see how you feel in the morning. (Do it on a Saturday night, so if you feel great—well, you've still got all morning together.)

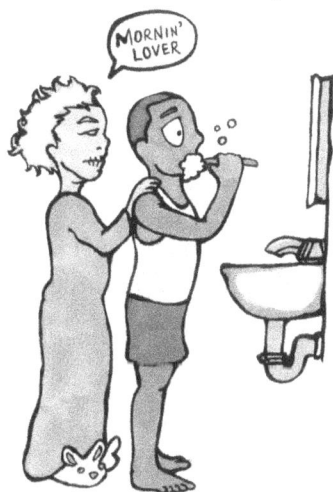

Do you know how your partner smells? Do you like it?

Yes, the way your partner smells—and your ability to talk to him or her about it—is really important. The cutest person in the world may have a body odor that really turns you off. The breath that smells so sweet at 8 p.m. may turn your stomach at midnight (or 8 a.m.!). And personal hygiene counts.

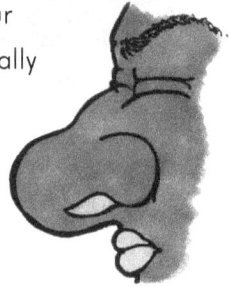

Good sex means really exploring someone's body. That's why it doesn't hurt to get to know someone *really* well before you have sex with them. And if you smell a body odor, you should be able to tell them about it.

If you can talk about body odor, then you know you feel pretty comfortable with your partner. It doesn't have to ruin the moment, either—try showering or taking a bath together. Not only will this guarantee that your partner's body is clean enough to touch and kiss all over; it's also a fun way for you and your partner to get to know each other's bodies.

Are you willing to walk around naked in front of your partner, with the lights on?

Sure you can have sex under the covers in the dark, so your partner never has to see your entire body naked. But if you don't feel comfortable showing your body to your partner, are you really going to enjoy having this person touch you and kiss you everywhere?

Most of us find it at least a little embarrassing to be naked in front of a new person at first. But sex can be really embarrassing, too. If you can't handle the naked part, maybe you're not really ready for the sex part.

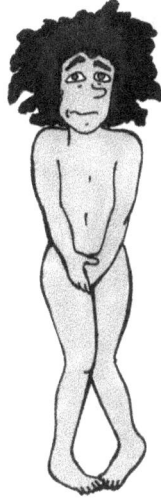

Have you gone as far as you can go before having sex?

It's tempting to jump straight to having sex, but going all the way is always better if you've fooled around a lot first. You want to feel comfortable and relaxed with each other, not shy or embarrassed. You want to know what makes you excited and what makes your partner excited. To get to that place you need to take the time to explore each other's bodies and experiment with each other. It will help the two of you figure out what you really like—and what you don't like.

Sex is going to feel a lot better (and you and your partner are going to feel a lot more comfortable with each other) if you build up to it gradually. So kiss, hug, lick, rub, and caress each other. You don't even have to take your clothes off. And don't be afraid to speak up. Say, "That feels good," or "I like that," or "That hurts," or "Not so rough," or "Stop."

If you reach a place in your relationship where you're having intercourse, keep on communicating with your partner. Let them know what you like and don't like. If you tell them what you want and how it makes you feel, sex will keep getting better. And you'll also learn how much your partner cares about you and your feelings. If you're with someone who only cares about his (or her) own pleasure and not yours, this is probably not the right person for you.

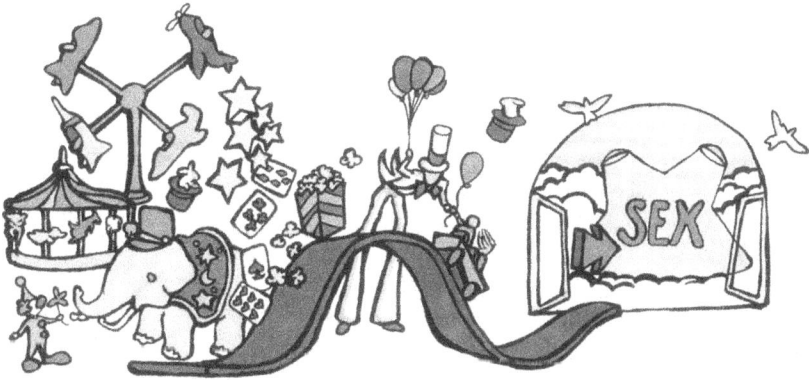

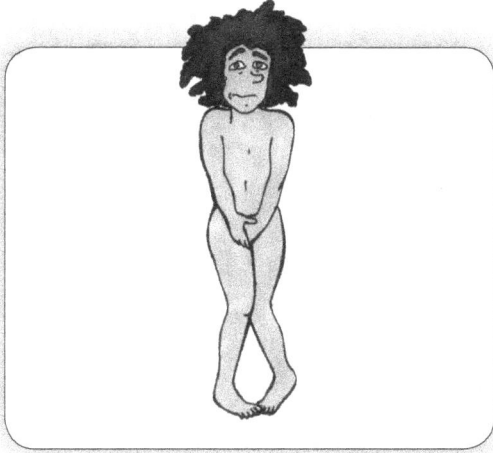

Getting Physical Without Sex

Teens Share Their Experiences

There's More to Sex Than Sex

By Loretta C.

Humping, fingering, jerking off, rubbing, petting, licking, sucking, stroking, first base, second base, third base, foreplay, kissing, hugging, necking, making out...Call it what you want, there is a whole other world outside of sexual intercourse.

"People do a lot of crazy stuff before they do it," said David, 17.

But why not do the crazy stuff *instead* of doing "it"? Especially if you don't have a condom, you're afraid of AIDS, pregnancy, or nasty things like genital warts—or if you're just not ready.

People often overlook things like kissing, hugging, even holding hands. "Anything can be erotic and enormously satisfying," said Andy Humm of the Hetrick-Martin Institute. "Sex is more than intercourse... It's more than doing the deed: the thing is in, the thing is out."

Humm recommends that teens use their imaginations. There are many ways of expressing yourself sexually other than intercourse.

"Humping" is about the closest you can get without putting yourself or your partner at significant risk of catching a sexually transmitted disease (STD) or getting pregnant. That's when two people rub their pelvic areas together simulating intercourse but the penis does not penetrate the vagina. It can be done with or without your clothes on. People also use their hands to stroke, finger and "jerk" each other. This is also known as mutual masturbation.

There are still some small risks that come with these alternatives.

Even without having intercourse you or your partner can contract chlamydia, herpes, or pubic lice (crabs), for example, just through genital contact. Any cuts, open sores or conditions such as poison ivy might pose a small risk because they are potential passageways for HIV infection.

One thing that's not safer than vaginal intercourse is anal sex. There have been studies claiming that about 25% of all teenagers have engaged in anal sex, often to avoid pregnancy or preserve their virginity. But anal sex is not a safe alternative since there is a higher risk of catching HIV, even with a condom. During anal sex, there is a greater chance that the condom will break and that tissue will tear. This can happen even if you don't see any blood.

The risks of STDs and unwanted pregnancy can be avoided if you choose an alternative to intercourse. One teen we interviewed said he has done some "other stuff" because he didn't have a condom. But he adds: "If we had a condom, we would have done it."

Other people who might not be ready for intercourse, might be ready for some of the alternatives. But not everybody is ready for what experts call "outercourse" either. "You have to ask yourself, 'Can I handle this?'" says Teri Lewis, director of the AIDS and Adolescents Network of New York.

Some people can't trust themselves; once they get started, they can't stop themselves after a certain point. Still others won't engage in any type of sexual activity until they are married. "There's no rush," said Ana, 17.

You have to decide for yourself what you think is right for you. Whether you choose to have intercourse, outercourse, or to remain abstinent, the most important thing is to talk about the decision with your partner.

There might be a point where you would like to stop. Say you don't want to do anything beyond French kissing, for example. According to Lewis, the two of you have to work that out together—ahead of time: "You have to decide that 'We won't get further.'"

But what if your partner disagrees with you? "Ask yourself the hard question, 'Is this the relationship that I want?'" Lewis cautions. "If you can't reach compromises about this then you probably can't reach others."

Loretta was in high school when she wrote this story.
She later graduated from college and worked in nonprofit marketing.

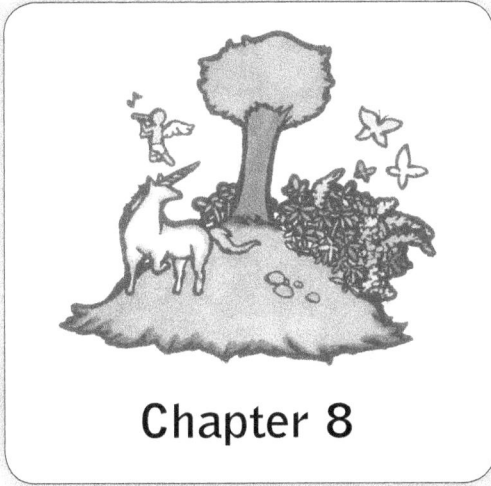

Chapter 8

Five Things to Ask About Where, When, and How

What's your first time fantasy? What's your partner's?

When they imagine what their first sexual experience will be like, most people have big dreams. Maybe they picture an ideal setting—a king-size bed in a fancy hotel or a deserted beach at sunset. Maybe they hear a mental soundtrack of music that they know will put them in the mood. Maybe there are magic words they can hear their partner say: "I love you," or "You're so beautiful," or "I've never felt this way about anyone before."

They probably have a few nightmare scenarios as well: girls worry that it will hurt so much that they won't enjoy it; guys worry that they'll come too fast (or not at all) and be humiliated; both guys and girls picture their parents walking in on them.

One way to make the actual experience more like the dream and less like the nightmare is to discuss your hopes and fears with your partner *before* you reach the point of no

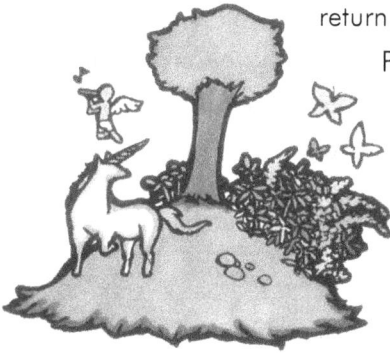

return. Even if you can't fly away to Paris or Tahiti for the weekend, you can still make it special for each other. And you can eliminate potential sources of anxiety. What's going to help you relax and enjoy yourself? Privacy? Physical comfort? A romantic setting? Having contraception handy? Time to talk and snuggle afterwards? Does your partner feel the same way?

And remember: even the best-laid plans aren't foolproof. Don't let your desire to make it special put too much pressure on yourself or your partner. Your first time may hurt a little, you may get a little embarrassed, and it probably won't look or feel much like the sex scenes you see in movies. But sex, like most things in life, gets better with practice.

Do you have a private place to have sex?

Sex is not a spectator sport. It's an intimate sharing between two people. If you have sex in a public place (or a semi-public place) like an unused room at school, a park, or the back seat of a parked car, there is always the possibility that someone will walk in on you unexpectedly (maybe with a video camera).

Of course, it's not always easy for teenagers to find a private place. But you should make every effort to find a spot where you and your partner can be alone without having to worry about being interrupted. You'll probably feel more relaxed and more able to express yourself freely.

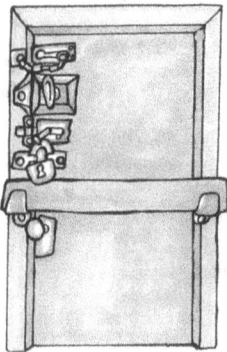

Will you have enough time?

Some people are fine with a quickie. Usually it's when a couple has known each other for a long time and had good sex for a long time. Then having a quickie—just to change the routine, or because they're both really sexually excited but don't have time for a long, romantic evening—can be pleasurable.

But generally speaking, taking your time makes sex much more pleasurable and rewarding. There's a reason why people like to give each other massages, or kiss and caress (it's called foreplay). Good sex is both a physical and emotional experience. It's not something most of us can just turn on and off like a switch. You need to build up to it and then come down from it. Having a quickie when it just feels rushed can leave you feeling unsatisfied, depressed, and even used. Don't get pressured into doing it if it doesn't feel right to you. Give yourself the time you need to make it the experience it should be.

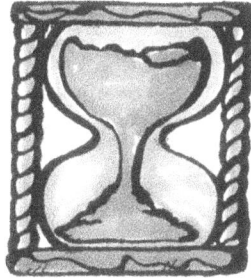

Will you have a chance to talk afterwards?

No matter how often you have sex or how many times you've done it, you always want to talk about your feelings afterward. Talking afterwards is part of sex. Many people find that in the hour or so after sex, they talk more openly and laugh more freely. They feel an intimate connection to their partner at that time that makes it easier for them to talk about things that might be difficult to bring up other-wise. It's also a time when people find it easy to just be silly with each other. So take advantage of the special closeness you feel after sex by sticking around and having a conversation.

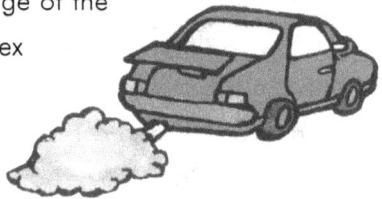

Have you imagined how you'll feel afterwards?

You've probably imagined your first experience of doing "it" dozens of times. Now jump ahead and imagine what happens next. Do you fall asleep in your partner's arms? Stay up all night together, whispering and giggling? Or do you throw your clothes on and get out of there fast, like you're fleeing the scene of a crime? Do you imagine being happy, relaxed, relieved? Or do you think you'll feel embarrassed, ashamed, anxious, guilty?

You should feel good while you're having sex, and you should also feel good about it afterwards. Sure, it's normal to worry about things like pregnancy, even if you've used every form of birth control under the sun. It's also common to feel strong emotions after having sex, not just love but also vulnerability. That's because sex is a big deal. (If it wasn't, we wouldn't have written this whole book about it.) But if you imagine that your first time will be followed mainly by fear or regret, maybe you should wait a little longer—for the right time and the right partner.

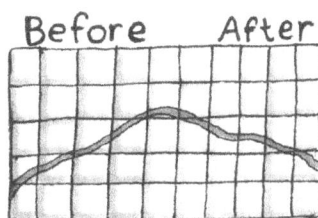

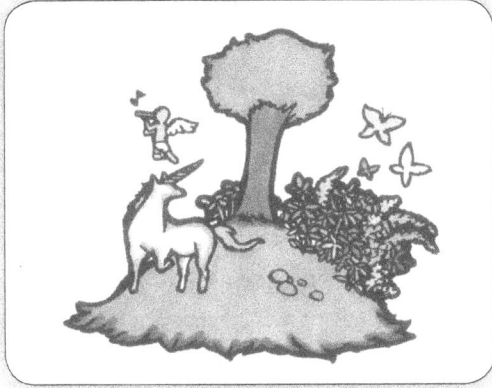

What to Expect

Teens Share Their Experiences

The First Time

By Jasmin Urias

Before our first sexual experience we all fantasize once in a while (come on, you know you have) about what we want it to be like or what we expect it to be like, based on what we've heard from our friends or seen on TV and in the movies. Some people dream about a beautiful, romantic experience and others worry that it's going to hurt or be embarrassing or that they just won't know what to do.

I thought it would be interesting to find out more about what teens think sex is going to be like and whether the reality is as good (or bad) as they thought. I decided to interview a bunch of people, guys and girls, virgins and non-virgins, to find out.

I started by asking people about their expectations. Not surprisingly, guys and girls tended to have different ideas about what having sex would be like and when they should start having it.

Like most guys I interviewed, Stephan, 17, expected it to be great. "I had imagined something strange that would make me feel damn good— long, sweet, and just all that," he said.

Mauricio, 19, also had high expectations. "I imagined it would be something beautiful, out of the ordinary," he said.

Although most of the girls I interviewed also dreamed about a first time that would be "beautiful" and "romantic," they also expected it to be less than perfect. As Catalina, 19, said, "I hope it would be romantic, but at the same time I know it's going to be hard, because I know I'm going to be very nervous since it's going to be my first time."

Alex, 15, said things people have told her about what the first time will be like have made her think twice about having sex. Some say it's a good feeling, but "others tell me it hurts," she said. Tiger, 16, also said her image of sex was influenced by what others said. "I expected it to be boring, since everybody told me it was," she said.

Before it happens, girls also tend to be more concerned about finding the right time, the right place and, especially, the right person for their first sexual experience. Beth, 15, said she's "waiting for the right guy, or somebody worth giving my virginity to." Alex is waiting, too, "till I get married, when I find the right guy."

Guys tend to be more eager to just do it; who they're going to do it with is not such a big concern. Kevin (not his real name), 18, spoke for a lot of guys I interviewed when he said, "It didn't matter, if it happened, it happened. If I had the chance, I'd go for it."

Almost all the teens I interviewed said they think people are in too much of a hurry to have sex.

But sometimes a guy's attitude will change after he meets someone special. Billy, 18, said, "When I used to think about my first time, I always used to say, 'I can't wait to get laid.'" He felt that way because "all my friends got laid and I didn't want to feel left out, I wanted to be part of the group." But then he met his current girlfriend and had a change of heart. They fell in love and he knew he wanted to lose his virginity to her.

Billy and his girlfriend were together for more than a year before they had sex. "I realized with [her] that it was something worth waiting for; it was something we both wanted to be special and have some meaning." He said the first time was scary because he didn't know what to do, but also "great and perfect...probably better than I thought it would be. Making love is something very special and nothing else compares to it." (Isn't he sweet?)

Billy isn't the only romantic guy out there. Mauricio also waited for someone special to have his first sexual experience with. He and his girlfriend had been going out for a year before they had sex. "I loved her a lot and she loved me, the relationship was going very well and I think that's why we did it," he said. "It was like a dream come true and it was beautiful."

Not every guy has as positive an experience as Billy and Mauricio did. For Stephan, who had been in a hurry to have sex because "what I had seen on the porno was quite interesting and tempting," the first time didn't come near to his expectations; it was just a big disappointment. What he and his partner actually did was nothing like what he "saw the pro do" in the porn film, Stephan said. "After those few minutes, when you come, it's like, what the hell is this?' and then you feel stupid."

For several of the girls I interviewed, the first time was better than they expected. Tiger, who had heard from her friends that sex was boring, got a pleasant surprise. "It was really fun," she said. Tiger had been dating her boyfriend for five years and even though they had spoken about having sex a couple of times, she didn't think he was "the one." Although she hadn't planned to do it, she said, "I think he planned it. The room was hot and there were rose petals and everything." (Rose petals, wow!)

Don't blow off something so important.

Kathy, 18, is someone else whose first sexual encounter was better than she expected. "It wasn't horrible, not at all," she said. The guy had been her best friend and then he told her that he loved her. "I was shocked. I told him he can't. I then fell in love with him. I love him till this day," Kathy said.

When I asked the people I interviewed if they had any advice for teens who hadn't had sex yet, Mauricio said, "I would tell all teens to go out and inform themselves about sex and its consequences, like pregnancy at such a young age, or even worse, STDs," he said.

For Tiger, the best thing about having sex with her boyfriend was that, afterwards, "We could talk about anything, we could tell each other everything." If you're thinking about having sex, she advised, "Talk about it with your partner, be open in the relationship."

Except for Kevin, who said, "Give it up whenever you have the chance. It's a good feeling," all the teens I interviewed said they think people are in too much of a hurry to have sex. Both guys and girls agreed that the most important thing was not to rush into it.

For Billy, the best thing about his first time was "that we waited so long, which made it so much more special. If we did it after a month or so, it would be OK, but since we waited more than a year, it made it beautiful." So his advice is, "Take your time, don't ruin the first time on somebody that won't matter to you in the future, make sure that person is special or it will be something you will regret."

To my surprise, Stephan agreed. He said he and his girlfriend had sex "at the wrong time" and he regrets it even though their relationship is good and they are still together. He said, "My only advice to teens is, don't get carried away with all the fine-looking and tempting stuff. Wait for the right time or you won't know what real love is."

Kathy had a similar point of view. "People should make it important," she said. "Don't blow off something so important."

Jasmin was 16 when she wrote this story.

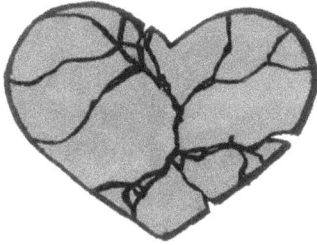

Chapter 9

**Five Things to Ask About
Dealing With the Consequences**

Are you ready for the intense emotions that can come with having sex?

Romantic feelings are usually intense, even when we're not having sex. That's because romance is all about our fantasies. Many of us fantasize about finding the kind of love that will make us feel like our whole lives make sense; like we've found our soul mate; like we've become the kind of person, and are with the kind of person, we've always dreamed of. Our romantic longings can be intense, and so can our fear of never finding love, or finding it and losing it.

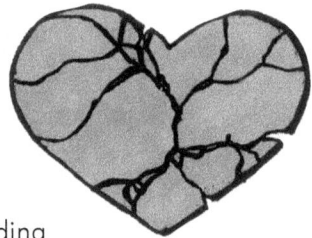

Then we throw sex into the mix. Now, some people can separate their romantic feelings from their sexual feelings, but many people cannot, even if they want to. They think they can have sex without becoming more attached to their partner, only to discover that they're not as in control of their emotions as they thought they'd be. Other people hope sex will make them feel the kind of connection and intensity they've been longing for. When they do, that intensity can feel wonderful, but it can also feel scary.

Before you have sex, ask yourself, am I ready for so much emotional intensity, or would it be too much too soon? Instead of improving my relationship, would it make me want to run away and ruin a good thing? Or make me so scared of losing my partner that I'd become jealous all the time, or always insecure?

Before you have sex, think about whether you're ready for the emotional intensity that can come with it. If you're not sure you are, take your time. There'll be other opportunities.

Could you and your partner recover from an awkward or unpleasant sexual experience?

The truth is, it's not always like in the movies, even if you know everything about your partner, from her favorite color to what he's most afraid of. Even if his (or her) kisses drive you wild, you've paraded around in front of each other naked, and have gone as far as you can go without having sex, it can still feel weird. Sometimes he comes too quickly. Or it hurts too much to continue. Or you get scared in the middle and want to stop.

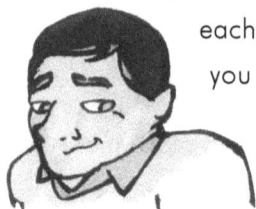

That's when you want to know that it's OK to be awkward. So ask yourself: Could you laugh about it, talk about it, and hold hands and hang out after, even if it is awkward?

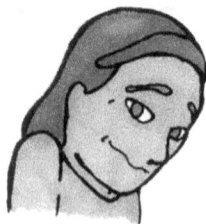

Could you handle being broken up with or falling out of love?

Breakups aren't easy. When they happen, we feel alone, angry, betrayed, depressed, sometimes even like our world is ending. And when we've had sex, the end of intimacy can feel even more devastating.

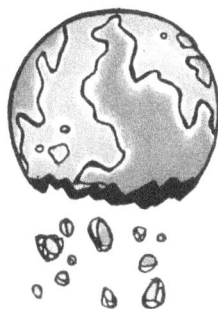

Usually, after time and effort—sometimes a lot of time and a lot of effort—we recover. We discover moments, even whole days and weeks, when we feel happy again. But if your partner's the only meaningful person in your life, and if the time you spend with him (or her) is the only time that you enjoy, then becoming even closer by having sex can be risky. You might be too devastated if the relationship ends. You might also be too likely to stay in a relationship that's hurting you.

If that's the way you feel right now, maybe sex isn't the answer. There may be some harder work you need to do first to feel better about your life.

Have you thought through what you'd do if you got pregnant?

The chances of you or your partner becoming pregnant are greatly reduced if you plan ahead and have safer sex. But even when you take all the proper precautions, pregnancy is still a possibility. That's why you shouldn't have sex unless you've thought deeply about abortion, adoption, and parenting, and taken time to imagine yourself facing those possibilities.

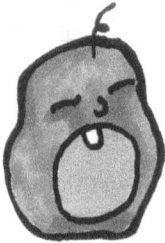

Many teens have no doubt that if they became pregnant, abortion would be the right choice for them. But sometimes they find out that when they do become pregnant, the decision to have an abortion is harder than they'd thought it would be. They feel a sense of loss or guilt, even though they know they're not ready to become parents yet. On the other hand, many teens who think that they would never have an abortion end up getting one after an unplanned pregnancy, and feel relieved about their choice.

Some teens know that if they or their partner got pregnant, they'd want to have the child. Then when they face the real possibility of parenthood, they change their minds. Or they do become parents, only to find the demands of parenthood more daunting than they ever imagined. They wish they had thought some things through more clearly before they started having sex, like: How will I support my child? Where will we live? Who will help me out when I need to go to school or work, or when I'm dying for a break or, just need to sleep? Do I have the emotional maturity and stability to parent a child?

It's not possible to know exactly how you'll feel until you're in the situation. But it is possible to talk to the people you know—and who you trust to tell it to you straight—about their own experiences with abortion, adoption, or parenting. Then take some time to imagine yourself in their shoes. If you can't imagine facing any of the options, maybe you ought to wait before having sex.

How would you handle it if you got an STD?

A lot of teens who get an STD say they thought they weren't the kind of person to ever get one—which is one of the reasons why too many teens don't do a thing about protection, and nearly 1 out of every 4 sexually active teens has an STD. But sometimes, even when you've done everything you're supposed to do, something unexpected happens. The condom breaks, or your partner, who says he's been monogamous, hasn't been.

Before you start having sex, it's good to ask yourself what you'd do if you did catch an STD. Would you know where to go to get treated? Would you be comfortable enough with your partners to tell them they also might have an STD? Would you be able to handle the emotional fallout from it, like how it might affect your relationships? Would you have people to turn to or would you be too scared or ashamed to ask for help?

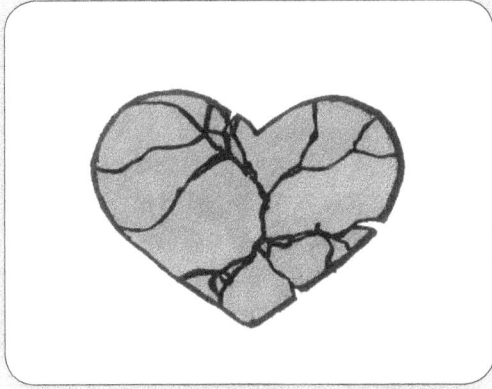

The Morning After
Teens Share Their Experiences

Am I the Father?

By Anonymous

One day in June, I received a phone call from a female acquaintance. We were having a normal conversation until she came out of nowhere and said, "I'm pregnant and I think it's yours." My eyes opened wide, and I asked her when this happened. "Remember back on October 2?" she said. "We did something."

I was stunned as I remembered what she was talking about. Then I couldn't think too well because anger came over me. I asked in a loud tone of voice, "How long did you know this? How many months are you?"

She told me that the baby was due next week and I was the father. I was furious. She had known this for nine months and was telling me only a week before the baby was due. I hung up on her.

I sat there trying to get my thoughts together. I knew the time she was talking about. In October, I was chilling and getting drunk at a party and I saw her across the room. I approached her and asked how she was doing. She said, "I've been eyeing you all night, and was waiting for you to come to me."

I was amazed. I thought, "Oh, really? Damn. That means I don't have to do that much." We went upstairs where the music wasn't so loud so we could talk alone. She told me that her name was Melanie and she didn't have a man but she was looking for one.

I said I was looking for someone too. That was a lie. Really I did have a woman, but I figured what she didn't know wouldn't hurt her.

Melanie started telling me about her life. She said her moms was a pain in the behind. She had an older brother who didn't care too much about her. I was kinda interested in her little tale. She said, "Let me get your number and we can talk on the phone sometime." I saw nothing wrong with that. She was cool enough and cute.

Then next thing I knew she started to fall asleep next to me. I tried to wake her up, and she pulled me towards her. We stared in each other's eyes for a hot second, and before I knew it she was kissing my cheek. So, me being drunk and she being drunk, we did our thang.

I felt weird after we had sex. I hadn't had a one-night stand before. I felt I straight up took advantage of her, and that seemed strange. After we were done, I left her and we never spoke again. But we kept hearing about each other through mutual friends. I just thought of her as a female I met at a party.

But now she had called me, nine months later, telling me a baby had come out of that night and that it would be in the world in a week. I felt very confused. I wanted to punch something.

Instead, I called my girl, who I had only recently started seeing, and told her what was going down. My lady sounded stunned on the phone but helped me think through the situation.

We both thought that the first thing I needed to do was to take a paternity test to see if the kid was really mine. We weren't ready yet to think too far beyond that. I kept asking myself, "What if it is mine? Am I ready to be a father? Am I ready to take care of another life?"

But I did know that if it was mine, I wasn't going to abandon it. I've seen too many fathers leave their kids behind. In fact, my own father left me behind when he went to jail. I knew the pain of growing up without a dad, and I always swore I wouldn't do that if I had a child. So I knew if I became a father, my teenage life was gone. I would have to stop acting like a boy and take care of my responsibilities as a man.

I didn't know what that meant, exactly. I didn't know whether it meant I would have to quit school to get a full-time job. I did know I was too young for this. What's worse, I didn't have a penny to my name. But the baby would need things: diapers, a crib, toys, clothes, milk.

So many thoughts in my head, so many things to do, and the way I saw it was I didn't have much time to do those things. The walls were closing in quick and I felt I had no one to help me.

I couldn't go back to selling products on the street. What good would I be to my kid if I were dead or locked up? I couldn't go to my parents—they would kill me. How the hell could I tell my moms that I had a kid? How could I tell any of my family members? I felt ashamed. I was supposed to be the one who succeeded, who didn't get caught in situations like this.

> **How was I ever going to handle getting along with the kid's mother, someone I couldn't stand for putting me through this?**

The only thing I knew was that I wanted to stay with my girl and I wanted to be part of this kid's life. No matter what the circumstances were, I wasn't leaving my seed. But how was I ever going to handle getting along with the kid's mother, someone who would be there in the kid's life forever, someone I couldn't stand for putting me through this?

Melanie called me back and asked why I hung up on her. I told her, "You knew all this and held out on me for this long, and you're wondering why I'm being mean to you? I want nothing to do with you. I want to be with my lady and that's it. The only reason I am going to be nice to you and show some respect towards you is for the kid."

I knew I was half responsible for all this and that made me even more mad.

At the time it was around graduation, and I had to pass the tests I needed to graduate. As I was studying for the tests and, later, taking them, my mind was on the baby. I could think of nothing but the baby, my girl, my family and how was I gonna make money.

For a while I thought that my girl would leave, too, for the simple fact that females hate dealing with baby mama drama. Still, she continued to stand by me.

"Why would I leave?" she said when I told her what I was afraid of. "I said I was going to be there for you and that's what I'm doing."

My friends who I told about the baby situation were shocked about the news, but they supported me 100%. I couldn't ask for better friends in a time of need.

But that didn't mean everything was good. I was nervous just thinking about becoming a father, and even with the best friends and girl in the world, I wasn't ready.

I had an idea of how hard it is to be a good parent. After all, neither of my parents pulled it off well enough to keep me at home, and I ended up in foster care. It hurt that my father had always been in and out of my life.

So when I'd thought of having kids myself, I wanted everything to be perfect. I wanted to have two, a boy and a girl, or as I would call them, my prince and princess. I pictured having my kids by the wife I chose to marry and that I would be financially stable enough to take care of them. Not to have everything completely the opposite — to have a kid by someone who I don't care for, and to raise a kid when I'm not stable.

> **I had an idea of how hard it is to be a good parent. After all, neither of my parents pulled it off well enough to keep me at home.**

On Thursday, June 20, Melanie had the baby. She called me two hours after she delivered and told me that it was a boy. I was happy to hear that it had gone well with her and that the baby was healthy.

I went to the hospital that Friday to take the paternity test. As he took some blood for my DNA, the doctor said the results wouldn't be ready for a few days. I felt weird having the blood drawn; my arm was flinching as he did it. I couldn't stop thinking about how all of this was happening so fast.

Afterward I went to see the baby. He was sleeping and beautiful. The last time I saw a baby that beautiful was when my lil' sister was born. I asked the nurse, "Could I hold him?" and she gave me the baby.

I sat there holding Shorty in my arms like a prized possession. I started talking to the baby like I already knew he was mine. He was cute, with hazel eyes, a little hair, and little hands and feet.

When the nurse told me that she had to put him back in the crib, I didn't want to let him go. The whole feeling that the baby was mine hit me hard. I saw Shorty's eyes and I knew that I would be ready for this. He was my responsibility and I wouldn't let him down.

The whole time I was in the hospital room, Melanie and I didn't communicate. The only time we spoke was when it regarded the baby. I told Melanie, "My only plans are to raise that baby, nothing else." She said she understood that.

I told her I would get the diapers and some toys, though I still hadn't figured out how. She said she and her mother would supply the clothes and the crib and I could see the kid whenever I wanted. I said I'd see Shorty after school and some nights that I had free. Melanie's moms was in the hospital, too. She seemed to like me, but she was also mad at me because she knew that we were too young and that we weren't ready for this.

Monday was the big day, the day I'd find out if the kid was really mine. At the end of the day, I was supposed to meet my lady and tell her the results.

When I got to the hospital, I saw Shorty moving, and I asked if I could hold him while the doctor went and got the results. So I sat there in a chair holding Shorty in my arms, rocking back and forth.

I started talking to him, telling him, "Hey, little one, I might be your father," and, "Don't worry, I will never leave you." I knew I was getting a little too mushy with Shorty, but I couldn't help it. I even felt the urge to cry and let some feelings out. The way the baby moved in my arms was a joyous feeling to me. He was lying there sleeping, eyes closed, his little fists tight. I couldn't believe he was mine.

After a while, Melanie caught my attention. She was just outside the room, and I saw that she was crying. Her mother got up and started yelling at the doctor, "It has to be him." I walked toward them, and as the yelling got louder, the baby started crying and the nurse took him away.

Melanie's mother told the doctor, "I'll pay you to tell him he is the father." I couldn't believe what I was hearing. I felt like I was about to flip out on her.

As I struggled to stay calm, the doctor pulled me to the side and told me eye to eye, face to face, that the child wasn't mine. I felt strange—both sad and overjoyed. I knew I wasn't ready to be a father, but I had been liking the idea of having a kid to call mine.

That night, I told my girl the news. She was glad. But later as I walked down the streets, I noticed all the babies who were with their fathers, and I started to miss Shorty. It was strange, all I'd been through in the last week because of that one-night mistake with Melanie. It was stranger to think that I could've been a father.

I had pictured having my kids by the woman I chose to marry, and that I would be financially stable enough to take care of them.

I call Melanie up once in a while to check up on Shorty. See how he's holding up. I was mad at her for doing all that to me, but I came out all right and she is having to give up her teen years.

To be honest, I believe some good has come out of it for me. My lady and I are stronger as a couple after going through that together, and I'm much more cautious about sex. Let's just say I always use a condom. I know that having kids isn't my thing, not now. (Maybe when I am about 22 and financially stable, I'll think about it.)

After seeing Shorty and holding him in my arms, I understand the love fathers have for their kids. But I also see why so many run. It's frightening to look at something so small and know how much he needs you. But that doesn't make it right for fathers to leave.

The author was 19 when he wrote this story.

Abortion Was the Right Choice for Me

By Lakia H.

Growing up in foster care, I lived in several homes with teenagers who became parents. The teen mom I remember best was only 16 when she had her first child, and was getting ready to turn 18 when she had her second. The only people she could depend on were her social workers, and sometimes not even them. She had no family and the fathers of her children did very little to help her. She was very much alone, struggling to raise her kids.

I swore that I was going to be nothing like her. I was going to finish school and get a job before even considering having a child. I had never been in a relationship with a guy, so I figured that getting pregnant at an early age would not happen to me.

Then, shortly after my 14th birthday, I began going out with a boy for the first time. He was friends with some of my friends, and older—he was 17. We had an off-and-on relationship that didn't involve sex, at least not for the first couple of years. Most people assume that being in a relationship as long as ours without sex would take a huge toll on the guy. Even I kind of thought that if I didn't eventually give him some, he'd leave me. Soon after I turned 16, we said that we loved each other for the first time and decided to start a sexual relationship.

At first I didn't think that having sex was going to change our relationship, but after a while it did. I think because I lost my virginity to him, it brought us closer together, even though, as far as I'm concerned, sex isn't all that it's cracked up to be. See, I let TV and movies influence my thoughts about sex. They make it seem like it's this wonderful thing, and that it's all glamorous. Sure, it's OK, but it's also very weird. It feels funny, the positions are funny, and it even smells funny. I don't understand why people exaggerate about it so much.

Anyway, my boyfriend and I didn't really talk about it, but we ended up using condoms for birth control. I had never taken any sex education classes, but we just had the common sense to know that protection was the best thing for both of us. So every time we'd have sex, we used a condom. Except for one time.

Summer started. Things were going well between my boyfriend and me. Then, I began to notice some changes in my body. I thought it was because of stress, but decided to go to the doctor anyway. That's how I found out that I was three weeks pregnant. I didn't expect to hear that—my period was only a day late. When the doctor told me the news, I thought she was joking. I started laughing. She gave me this look and said, "Seriously, you're pregnant."

I still didn't believe it, not until she gave me some information about abortion and adoption. She told me to read it and come back in two weeks with a decision. I had to decide whether to keep the baby, have an abortion, or have the baby and give it up for adoption. This would become the hardest two weeks of my life.

When I told my boyfriend I was pregnant, he was more shocked than I was. He asked me what I wanted to do, and for some strange reason I said I wanted to get an abortion, even though I wasn't really sure. It just seemed like the logical thing to say. My boyfriend didn't have any objections. He said I should think of my future, which was true, since most likely I would be the one raising the child.

Then, the next weekend, I saw a show on TV called *Eclipse of Reason*. It showed actual footage of a woman getting an abortion, and included interviews with two women who said they were hurt mentally and physically from having abortions. By the end of the half-hour, my stomach was turning and I was in tears. The program led me to believe that if I went through with an abortion, I was a bad person. So my mind was set: I wasn't going to get an abortion. I felt as if I had made a big decision, but reality would soon wake me up.

I still looked through the bunch of papers that I got from my doctor and some other stuff I got from the Internet about abortions. What I read was very different from what the TV show said. The information from my doctor and the Internet reported that the mental and physical complications from abortion are extremely rare. I now think the TV show was created not to give an accurate account of abortion, but only to persuade women not to have them.

I began thinking of the teen moms I knew, and especially those whose kids later ended up in foster homes without them.

I began thinking of the teen moms I knew, and especially those whose kids later ended up in foster homes without them. I realized that *Eclipse of Reason* showed women getting abortions, but it didn't show young women struggling to raise kids alone, with no money, no support, and no job.

I began to think about all the things I wanted to do with my life that would be hard to do if I had a baby. I wouldn't be able to go to college full-time. If I found the time to get a job, I wouldn't get to keep the money for myself. I would have to buy baby clothes, milk, and diapers, and pay for a babysitter just to leave the house.

And having a kid at my age would not just be unfair to me, it would be unfair to the child, who would grow up without stability. He or she would be subjected to an unprepared mother and an environment where nothing is certain. The child would have to deal with the stress of having her mother struggle and do her damnedest just to keep a roof over our heads and food in our stomachs. I suspected I would make a good mother someday, when I had a steady job and a roof over my head. I also knew that now wasn't that day.

But I still didn't want an abortion. The thought of it was scary, and I wondered if it was wrong. So I thought briefly about adoption, but didn't like the idea of carrying something for nine months and becoming bonded to it as it got big, and then having to give it away. So instead of deciding what to do, I didn't decide. My two week deadline to go back to the doctor and to let her know what I wanted to do passed. Finally, I realized time was running out.

The day I decided to call Planned Parenthood to arrange for an abortion was the longest day of my life. I tried calling from the time I woke up until about 1 p.m. When I finally got through I told them that I wanted to make an appointment. The woman on the other end asked for what, and for some reason the word "abortion" would not come out of my mouth. When I finally said it, she gave me a date to come in: the next day. I had been hoping to have a couple of days to collect myself before having the operation.

The next morning my foster mother and my boyfriend went with me to the doctor. When I got there, I saw many women of all different ages, all waiting to have an abortion. One girl I met was 14 and was also having her first abortion. Another woman was 30 and already had two kids and had had two abortions before. We passed the time talking and watching TV.

> I suspected I would make a good mother someday, when I had a steady job and a roof over my head. I also knew that now wasn't that day.

When I finally made it into the operating room, I lay on the table. After that, all I remember is praying to God, asking Him to let me make it through OK. About 20 minutes later I woke up and started crying. Then I went home. All day, as I dealt with the physical aftermath of the abortion—mostly bleeding and cramps—I thought about my decision. I pictured myself with and without a baby. I thought about whether I was going to go to hell or not because of the abortion.

To this day, almost a year later, I still think about what my life would have been like with a baby. For one, I probably would be raising it alone, because my boyfriend and I broke up, though we're still friends.

For another, I probably wouldn't be going away to college this fall. And though sometimes I still have mixed feelings about abortion, for the most part I'm glad I made the decision to have one.

Not too long ago I was looking through the *TV Guide* and saw that *Eclipse of Reason* was coming on again. I thought about the message that show was trying to get across—that abortion was evil and that it would scar a woman for life if she had one. I think it's irresponsible to just say that abortion is bad without also showing how hard it is to raise a child before you're ready.

Yes, it's a bad idea to become pregnant when you aren't ready to be. And people should do everything they can to prevent unwanted pregnancies. But I think abortion only becomes bad when women see it as something as simple as brushing their teeth in the morning. If they say, "Oh well, I'm pregnant again, I'll just get an abortion," they're using it as a form of birth control, and I think that's wrong. But once a woman is pregnant, she is the one who should decide what to do, because she is the one who will live with her decision. And believe me, making that decision is hard enough without people telling you what to do.

Lakia was 17 when she wrote this story.
She later earned her GED and went to college.

My Sex Story

By Anonymous

When I was 16, my friends Sasha, Jasmine, and I made a bet over who'd lose her virginity first. We were the last holdouts in our larger group of friends.

I mainly thought my friends were too young to be having sex. Only recently, it seemed, we were playing with Barbie dolls, and now they were talking about all the sexual things they did and what they wanted to try out next. Still, I was the oldest one among my friends, and to hear them talk about having sex made me feel like I was younger than they were. I told myself, "If they can do it, why can't you?"

But then I'd think, "You're too young. Don't you want to wait until marriage? It'll be more romantic."

I'd go back and forth in my mind:

"There's so many people in the world; do you really think you're going to stay with one guy forever? Don't you want to see how other guys are?"

"That's how diseases spread."

"I'm not dumb."

"You are if you're thinking about having sex just to get it over with."

A couple of months before the bet, my friends and I had adopted a new phrase—"It's all for experience"—which I came up with because I wanted some adventure in my life. I heard a lot of people say the best way to learn is from experience, which I believe. So even though I was scared of sex, I entered the bet.

Having sex just for the experience seemed easier than trying to get into a relationship in order to have sex. I thought that maybe I could detach myself from the emotional part of sex so I wouldn't get hurt if we broke up. Besides, I was having problems at school and at home. I was depressed and longed to get rid of that feeling. I thought sex might help.

But I didn't have much opportunity to have sex. Then a year later, when I was 17, I met Chris.

We met in a hotel hallway in Georgia, at a friend's 21st birthday. As I walked my friend Kim to the elevator, she stopped Chris in the hallway and said, "Hey! Boy, doesn't she look fine?"

"Boy?!" said Chris. "I ain't no boy."

Kim looked at him and giggled, "You know what I mean... son!"

Chris smiled and said, "Yeah, she looks cute." I blushed and they started teasing me. Then Kim got in the elevator and Chris and I stayed.

I thought he was charming and cute—a beautiful smile, with dimples—and he was 6 feet tall, and built. I let my daydreams take over—of us being together for many years.

We talked for nearly two hours in the hallway about almost everything, including... sex. I even told him I was a virgin and that I would only do it with someone I loved. (I sorta stretched the truth.) He told me about his sexual experiences, including details I didn't need to know but was curious enough to ask about. He was three years older than I was, and wasn't a virgin. When I finally let him into my room, I suspected something big was going to happen.

What happened next was all a blur. I didn't understand why I didn't stop it. But it wasn't like I wanted to stop either, because I was curious and thinking to myself, "It's all for the experience." He closed the door, turned the TV way up, and things went on from there.

In the beginning, it was lovely. The kissing was fun, the caressing was nice, sweet, and romantic, but the initial you-know-what wasn't. Painful? Hell yeah!

We used a condom. I wouldn't have done it if he didn't have one, since I wasn't into catching an STD or getting pregnant.

So many things were happening at once and I felt a wave of emotions: "OH MY GOD, wake me up! Why am I here? I'm actually doing it. I want to call my friend. Is this how it's supposed to feel? I want to go home. I want him to love me." I knew that I'd changed, but didn't understand how.

Afterwards, he looked at me and smiled. I wanted to punch him in the face. I didn't feel good about what I'd done. I felt like a fool because I was with someone who was practically a stranger.

I wondered if it would have felt the same if I were with someone I knew and loved. I hadn't felt any real passion. And what was I going to do when I got home? Would I tell my mother? Could she find out just by looking at my face? Should I tell Kim and Sasha or keep it to myself?

"So what's up? Talk to me," he said.

Was he the slut, or was I?

I didn't want to talk to him. I didn't want to look at him. I hated him. I turned over and said that I was sleepy. I pretended to sleep, but I was thinking about the whole thing. I wanted to cry. I thought I had more respect for myself than to just do it with a stranger. Was he the slut, or was I?

Chris stayed in my room until 5 a.m., because we all had to leave by 7 a.m. to take the plane home after the celebration. I went into the shower hoping to wash off the feeling of failure. He tried to talk to me during the bus ride to the airport and on the plane, but I ignored him and sat with other people.

But I'd given him my number before we'd started fooling around, and once we got home, he called me persistently. I thought it was sweet the first time he called, but then I thought he was just being nice to me because he felt guilty, and I didn't want any of his sympathy. I was afraid to let myself feel romantic toward him, because then I'd be emotionally vulnerable. I was still all shook up from the things I remembered doing. I was so focused on the fact that I'd had sex, I was blind to the clues that he actually liked me. I just thought, "God, why doesn't this punk stop calling me?!"

Even my mother noticed I wasn't acting like myself. I was unusually quiet and wrote nonstop in my journal, recording every thought I had, trying to make sense of them since I wasn't talking to anyone about what had happened.

I didn't check my e-mails. I didn't even watch my favorite TV show. Mom would say, "Your show is on. You're not going to watch it? You're not going to check your e-mail? You've changed since you came back." I felt like telling my mother everything, but I couldn't, not yet. I needed to sort things out first.

Having sex just for the experience seemed easier than trying to get into a relationship.

Five days later, I decided to see Chris. My plan was to act like a real b-tch so he'd leave me alone. I didn't want to deal with the constant reminder of that night.

But when I saw Chris, I couldn't even look him in the eyes. We walked on the boardwalk and I was quiet the whole time. Then we went to see his friends. I was still quiet, but I laughed at his friends' jokes. He was sweet and respectful, talking to me calmly and wanting to know things about me. I realized that there was potential for a real relationship, so I decided to see him again.

Seven months later, Chris and I are boyfriend and girlfriend. I'm surprised that the first person I slept with became my guy. I always thought that it would be the other way around: He'd be my guy first and then later we'd be passionate together.

I've met his family, but he hasn't met mine yet. He wants to, but I finally told my mother that I'd had sex and she wasn't pleased, so Chris and I both think it's better to wait.

It's not simple though. We've broken up—and gotten back together—several times. My feelings have changed many times, very fast, from August till now. I hated him, liked him, was annoyed by him, bothered by him, loved him, hated him and loved him. He says that my fluctuating attitude is what bothers him the most about me.

Now that I'm in a relationship, I have a better sense of why I was afraid of relationships before, because the emotions can be overwhelming. When I love Chris, he's the best person in the world. But when I feel neglected because he has things to do, I hate him. When I have things to do, I think he feels bad too, because he'll say something stupid like "I think this is a sign." I hate that, because he makes it sound like neither of us is committed to the relationship.

But we're working on all that. This relationship is work, but I also think you have to work hard for some of the best things in life, like good grades. I've had sex with Chris since that first time. I enjoy it more now because I have this feeling of love inside me, rather than confused feelings for someone I just met.

I don't regret having sex because I don't think there was any other way of learning than through experience. But I wonder, would things between us be better if I had waited?

I think if Chris and I had only kissed that night, we'd still have gotten into a relationship, but we would've known a lot more about each other before we did something as dramatic as having sex. That would've been better since I might've been a little calmer starting our relationship, and we could've avoided a lot of arguments along the way.

The author was in high school when she wrote this story.

A Family to Raise Her

By Jennifer Olensky

It was as if all the glory of heaven was shining down, into my heart, my soul. In her eyes I learned the true meaning of love, in her presence the feeling of complete tranquility. This tiny miracle was the most beautiful child I had ever seen.

I cannot believe it has been 11 years since I said goodbye to my daughter. As I sit here looking at her picture, I think about how it all happened, and what led me to the choices I made.

Shortly after my 13th birthday, I went to live with my father. My father had always made me feel like "Daddy's little girl," showering me with love. But when I was 5, my parents separated and my dad disappeared for three years. At the time, I believed his absence was my mother's doing, and I embedded a hatred of her in my heart. I spent that time building my father up in my imagination. He was a king to me; he could do no wrong.

When I finally saw him again, my quest to live with him began. It led to bitter fighting between my mother and me, until the day she let go. When I arrived at Daddy's, I thought I had what I had wanted for so long.

I was wrong. My Daddy loved me, he told me so every day. The only problem was his need for pills and heroin. Often we did not have food to eat. Eventually he began beating me. Several times I thought I would die. By the morning he never remembered. I knew I had to leave, but I really had nowhere to go. My mother would hang up the phone upon hearing my voice, so I turned to my boyfriend, Alex. I was 14, he was 18. He snuck me into his house some nights. Not wanting to get him in trouble with his family, I would often sleep in his car.

Alex was all I had. He told me he loved me and I believed I loved him. For three months I clung to him for my life. Then the police picked me up. They brought me to a Catholic group home for girls. After my first physical, I was sent to Rosalie Hall, a home for pregnant teens. That was the way I learned that I was pregnant.

When I told Alex, he said that if I didn't get an abortion, he was washing his hands of the whole situation. But I never even considered abortion. I wanted a family. At the time I had no one, and I guess I needed something to hold onto. When Alex told me he wanted nothing to do with a baby, I was upset, but also in denial. I didn't believe that he would be so cold. I thought eventually he'd come around...but he didn't.

The 30 other girls in Rosalie Hall, the aides who spent most of the time with us, the teachers, counselors, cleaning lady, and even the cook welcomed me. They tried to be like family, but they were not. I had lost everything. I felt alone and scared.

Alex still insisted he loved me, which gave me something to hold onto. He kept in touch until I was about three months pregnant. Then he told me he couldn't continue to be in touch. He said it was only because he didn't want his family to find out I was pregnant with his baby. I was foolish enough to believe him.

For the next two months, I thought mainly about Alex. But after not hearing from him for all that time, I began thinking about my baby. The more I thought about it, the more I knew I needed to give my child a good life. The hardest part was realizing I could not. I was alone in the foster care system, but I wanted my child to have a loving, supportive environment with a mother and a father. At five months, I decided to give my child up for adoption. I told my counselor, Stephanie. We spoke about it several times. I knew deep within that it was right, but I decided not to tell anyone else. I knew the other girls would ridicule me, and the decision was hard enough already.

During the last few months of my pregnancy, Alex visited once and called twice. Each time he proclaimed his love for me. I believed all he said. I guess I needed to believe. Like with my father, in my eyes Alex could do no wrong. I spent every waking moment listening for the phone to ring, wishing he would call. Most nights I cried myself to sleep.

When I was seven months pregnant I met Ann, a social worker with the adoption agency. She came to visit me several times. I told her I wanted my baby to have a good life. She did her best to assure me that everything would be fine. Ann presented me with files of different families. Eventually I chose a couple who had been together several years. She was a college professor, he a lawyer. From their file, I felt confident that they had a strong sense of family, with a marriage built on mutual love and respect. I knew they were the ones.

I wanted a family. At the time I had no one, and I guess I needed something to hold onto.

On September 28, my labor started. On September 29, I arrived at the hospital at 9:30 p.m. I was alone, scared, and in a world of pain. Looking back with the faith I have now, I believe God was with me, not only in those final hours of my pregnancy, but every step of the way. I cannot understand where all my strength and energy came from if not from God.

On September 30, at 1:46 a.m., I looked into my daughter's eyes, and love, joy, and happiness overwhelmed me. In the midst of all life's tragedies my heart was singing. For the first time in my life, I felt true love. Over the next two days, I spent every possible moment with her. I never wanted to forget. I never wanted that feeling to fade.

Ann was supposed to pick her up on the third day. I was not ready to let go. I asked for three more days. Ann was reluctant at first, but gave in. The evening before I was released from the hospital, Alex came to see us. I had called to inform him of her birth. I suppose he wanted to satisfy his curiosity. He held her and fed her. When he said goodbye, he left in tears, never voicing his feelings. It was devastating. Part of me wanted him to say, "OK, we are going to keep her!" But I knew it would not happen.

For the next few days after I left the hospital, I was living close by so I walked over about four times a day to see my baby. She was extremely quiet; I never heard her cry. She would let out a small noise, then put her fingers in her mouth. She fussed a little when hungry, but as soon as she heard my voice, she became very quiet and alert.

Only a few days and I felt so connected. "How can I do this?" I thought. I asked Stephanie what would happen if I changed my mind.

"Foster care," was her response. "You did not apply for mother-child placement. There are waiting lists."

I thought about it and knew it would be wrong. She deserved an immediate warm loving environment, not the uncertainty I would face. Besides, I wanted her to have a permanent, stable home, and that was something I knew at the time I couldn't provide.

The morning Ann came to get her, I had time for one more feeding. As I held her, I spoke to her, studied, rocked, and hugged her. After some time I settled her into the bassinet and rubbed her back as she fell asleep. Kissing her head, I said goodbye. It was so hard to leave. I began to feel numb, just going through the motions, trying to stay strong. Then we went to Stephanie's office with Ann and Sister Diane, and I was presented with adoption papers. As they were explained to me, I sobbed, unable to stop. Sister Diane said, "That's it! I will not notarize these papers. You are keeping your baby." Then Ann put the pen in my hand. That shocked me, and suddenly I stopped crying and signed the papers. I quietly walked back to my room and stared at the wall.

In giving my baby up, I gave two loving people the family they longed for, her the chance to thrive, and myself the chance to grow.

I don't remember much of what happened over the next several days. As I slowly resurfaced, I thought and thought. The most important thing

I thought about was them—the couple, my daughter's parents. Instead of thinking about my loss, I was able to imagine their joy as they set their eyes upon their child. I shared in their happiness and trusted that they would take this truly amazing gift and nurture her, love her.

I have some pictures, and a five-page letter her parents sent me. In their letter, my daughter's parents said that I was their angel sent from heaven, that I was a special person with the capacity to love in a special way. They believed I had a wonderful future ahead, and that God always provides a time to be happy.

I also sent a letter to them and one for our daughter when she is older. I know I will see her one day, and hope to develop a relationship then. I know they are special people and that our daughter was the angel heaven sent. My future looks great, and God really does provide a time to be happy. I did what was right and do not regret it. In giving her up, I gave two loving people the family they longed for, her the chance to thrive, and myself the chance to grow, to become the person I am now. I think of her on a regular basis, she is a part of me. Although I cannot see her, the love for her in my heart continues to grow.

Jennifer was in high school when she wrote this story.

Teen Mothers Grow Up Fast

By Janice Brooks

When a teenage girl has a baby, it changes her life. She has to grow up quickly, because having someone else to take care of means taking on a lot of new responsibilities. In addition to taking care of her baby, she may have other problems to deal with—her family might throw her out of the house, her boyfriend might leave her, she might have to drop out of school. She ends up losing the fun and freedom of her teenage years because she can't just hang out and be a kid anymore.

"Being a mother comes with stress and responsibility," said Priscilla, 18, who has a 1-year-old son. "I have days that I want to go out and I don't have a baby sitter. Sometimes my baby gets sick and I can't go out. Sometimes I am too tired. I can't think about me anymore, I have to think about the baby."

When they heard the news that they were pregnant, the young women I interviewed felt a range of emotions. They were shocked, scared, confused, and embarrassed.

Two years ago, Samantha, 20, made a doctor's appointment because she thought she had the flu. It turned out that she was pregnant. "I was shocked," Samantha said. When the doctor told her the news, part of her felt happy, but she was also scared and confused. "Scared [because I] didn't know what the baby's father would say. Confused [because I] didn't know what to do about anything," Samantha explained.

Priscilla had a similar reaction when she found out that she was pregnant. "I was scared of my mother, scared of what the baby's father was going to say," she said. "I didn't know what to do."

Priscilla was right to be worried about what her mother and boyfriend would think. Her mother kicked her out of the house when she found out, forcing Priscilla to move into a shelter for pregnant teens. The baby's father wasn't there for her either. "I really didn't have a relationship [with him]," Priscilla said. "Every day of the week he had a different girl. He didn't care that I was pregnant."

When Crystal, 18, found out that she was pregnant, she knew that she wasn't ready to handle it. "I didn't know what to do," said Crystal, who was 14 at the time. "I was confused, there was a lot going on in my mind. I was a baby." One thing that's helped is that in her case, her daughter's father stayed involved. "Her father is definitely a daddy," Crystal said. "He loves her. He takes her out and takes great care of her. He has been a great father with her for the past two and a half years."

For many young women, getting pregnant doesn't just affect their relationships with their families and boyfriends, it also affects their friendships. Taurshia, 20, had a baby boy when she was 18. Taurshia said her friends were complaining about how their reputations were going to be ruined. "None of my friends from before are my friends now," Taurshia said.

Crystal said that she, too, lost one of her closest friends when she had her baby. "She stopped coming around as often because she didn't have nobody to party with," Crystal said.

On the other hand, some teen moms have friends who stick with them through their pregnancies. Their friends even help after the baby is born. Nelly, 19, had her baby when she was 15. At first, she was worried about how people would react. But her friends stood by and gave her a lot of support. "They love my baby boy as if he were their son," Nelly said.

But even with the help of friends and relatives, meeting their children's day-to-day needs is usually a struggle for teen moms. "Now I have to work two jobs," Nelly said. "I dropped out of high school. I have to think about my baby before thinking of myself."

"It's hard, it's very stressful," Priscilla agreed. "I have days that I can provide food and days that I can't." It's frustrating, Samantha said, because "working so much to get the money," she doesn't have enough time to spend with the baby.

But in spite of all the hard times, the teens moms I interviewed love their children with everything they've got.

"Being a mother is wonderful," Nelly said. "The best things are the hugs, kisses. It shows that he loves me a lot. He is the most important thing in this life. I would die for him. I just love him."

Taurshia said that it's a great feeling "having someone to teach and coming to you for guidance, knowing that all of the steps that I take or the decisions that I make will have an impact on his life."

But even though their children are so important to them, the young moms I interviewed don't encourage other teens to follow in their footsteps. All of them participate in a program called "Do as We Say, Not as We've Done," that advises teenage girls to put off having a baby.

"Being a mother comes with stress and responsibility," says one teen mom.

They tell younger girls how hard and how scary it was for them. They warn girls to be careful about sex—either not to do it too early or to use birth control.

"Getting pregnant changed my attitude about sex because now I am afraid to do it, and when I do, I always use condoms," Priscilla said. "What I would tell teenage girls about having sex is: if you're going to have sex, use condoms [and other forms of birth control] to help prevent you from getting STDs and unplanned pregnancies."

Taurshia advises girls to put off having children "until your financial status is stable and you are mentally stable and you are sure that this baby is something that you and the father are ready for."

Crystal said that having a child has forced her to grow up faster than she would have liked, but that it's been worth it because of the joy her daughter brings into her life. Like all the young women I interviewed, she's doing her best to make a good life for herself and her child.

"I am an adult and a kid at the same time," Crystal said. "My life is complicated, but I made it that way and all I have to do is keep it in control."

Janice was 16 when she wrote this story.
She went on to graduate high school and go to college.

My Boyfriend Lied

By Anonymous

Let me tell you about the day that changed my destiny. It was July 30, 1998. Ten days after I turned 20 years old. I was working for the Gay Men's Health Crisis, and excited about moving out on my own within a year.

Two weeks before, I had gotten tested for HIV. I started getting tested when I was 16 years old because I was having sex and sometimes didn't use a condom.

I had always gotten a negative result, meaning I didn't have HIV. And since the last time I'd been tested, the only person I'd had unprotected sex with was my long-term boyfriend. He assured me that he had been tested for HIV and that he did not have it. He refused to show me the test results, but I trusted him. He had been asking me to have unprotected sex for some time, and I eventually gave in. The condoms went out the window for the duration of our relationship.

After about a year and a half, our relationship ended. It wasn't long before I was over him and loving being single.

So back to July 30. In the waiting room, I thumbed through a magazine but I couldn't read any of the articles. I always felt a little anxiety waiting for the results of my HIV test. When it was time to go see what my results were, I said a prayer.

"Excuse me, Pedro?" a voice called out, interrupting my thoughts.

"Let's go into my office so we can have a little more privacy," the HIV counselor said.

She told me what the three possible test results were, the stuff you hear every time you get tested for HIV. It was either: negative, meaning I didn't have HIV; inconclusive, meaning the test was unable tell whether I had HIV and I would need to be tested again; or positive, meaning I had contracted HIV.

As she went on, I got more and more anxious. I really just wanted to know what the results were.

Then she told me what I would need to do if I was negative. "Be sure to continue practicing safe sex, get tested in six months, and be with only one partner," she said, sounding like a mother telling me to wear clean socks.

I tuned her out then because I didn't want to think about it.

"OK, and now for your results," she said.

"Ladies and gentlemen, the envelope please," I thought to myself.

She opened the file and placed it on her desk.

"Pedro, your results came back positive," she blurted.

The blood ran from my body. I was in shock. How? Why? But most of all, who? Who gave me HIV?

I swallowed and tried to compose myself. I kept telling myself to breathe. Why me? I was so young. I felt as if I had let down people who cared about me. I felt guilty for being gay. I felt like this was a punishment from God. I did everything possible to prevent myself from crying.

"Are you OK?" she was asking.

"Yeah, fine." It was a lie, of course.

"You might want to take a few days off to relax and absorb this. This is not going to be easy for you, but you can do it. Understand that this does not mean a death sentence."

Everything else she said was just a blur. I couldn't listen anymore. I needed to leave. I wanted to go home and crawl up in bed. I didn't want to think about this. Not now.

I went straight to my boss's office. I told her that I needed to leave immediately. She allowed me to take off the next two days. I went outside and walked around aimlessly for two hours.

I was angry, so angry. I didn't know what to do with myself so I tried calling my ex to tell him what had happened. I was confident that he was the one who infected me. By the time I got to his house, I was fuming mad. I wanted answers and I wanted them yesterday.

"How could you do this to me?" I asked.

"Who did you tell?" he wanted to know. He didn't want any of my friends getting revenge on him.

"What does it matter? I told those who are concerned about me."

"You shouldn't have done that. Why didn't you call me first? We could have handled this together."

"No, we couldn't have," I replied, getting more agitated by the moment. "Look, all I want to know is, are you positive?"

"Uh, yeah, I just got tested recently and I found out I was positive."

"You what?" My voice was getting louder and I was beginning to get choked up. I couldn't believe this was happening. "I think you've been positive longer than you say you have. How could

My boyfriend assured me that he had been tested for HIV and that he did not have it.

you do this? I asked you over and over if you were negative and you lied to me! What am I supposed to do now?"

"Listen, baby, we can work this out." He tried to pull me closer to him.

"Get off of me! There is nothing to work out!" I pulled away from him. I had heard enough. "F--k you! Don't ever bother me again!" I screamed. I was crying now. There was nothing more to say or do. I picked up my book bag, wiped my face with my shirt, and stormed out of his house. My head was pounding. I could hear him calling me to come back. I kept walking.

I went home and got in bed. I couldn't eat. I felt as if my life had stopped. I had so many emotions swirling in my head that I could not even think straight.

As I lay in my bed, I remembered all the people I already knew who were living with HIV. They were able to do everything they wanted to do in their lives. Nothing stopped them. Their sense of humor also helped them to deal with it. Remembering them made me feel a little calmer.

I knew I could talk to them about what I was going through. I also knew I had many other people who could help support me. I kept telling myself that I was fortunate to have tested positive in 1998 and not 1988, a time when little was known about HIV and there were very few medications available.

But I was also pissed off. Although the responsibility of deciding to have unsafe sex fell in my lap, I was angry because I had given my ex the benefit of the doubt. I had trusted him. And he had failed me. I felt like he took my life away from me.

I wanted to get even with him for lying to me. But deep inside, I knew that revenge would get me nowhere. Afterwards, I would still be HIV positive. Nothing could change that. I fell asleep hoping that when I awoke, this day would have been a dream.

After several weeks, once the initial shock wore off, I began looking for ways that I could improve my life, both physically and emotionally. I'd never allowed any challenge in my life to take me down before and I was not about to let this one be the first.

I began to go to therapy to help myself deal with being HIV positive. Therapy taught me that although I may be faced with a life-threatening illness, I shouldn't use it as a reason for not trying to achieve the things I want in life. In fact, it should be the reason for achieving the goals I want, such as finishing college and moving out of New York. I promised myself that I would not give up without a fight.

I started spending a lot of time alone, just looking at my life. If I wanted to live longer, I knew that I needed to spend more time on me and less time in the clubs. I needed to make sure that I got enough rest, reduced my stress, and took my medications.

Above all, though, I needed to practice safe sex at all times. I did not want to infect another person. I did not want to live the rest of my days knowing that I was responsible for that.

I went back to college soon after finding out that I was HIV positive. I wrote a final report, which was close to 175 pages, about learning to cope with HIV. Writing really helped me put what happened to me over the past year into perspective. It helped me realize how strong a person I really was. It also helped me find ways of coping, such as exercising, talking more with my friends, and getting acupuncture when life was getting too stressful for me.

I got an A+ on the paper and was the only student in my class to make it onto the dean's list that semester.

This past summer marked three years since I learned that I was positive. I am now working as the administrative director for a community foundation, and am still trying to finish that college degree.

I had trusted my ex, and he had failed me. I felt like he took my life away from me.

My viral load is undetectable, which means that the amount of HIV in my body is so low that the current available tests cannot detect it. It does not mean that I am negative, it just means that there isn't a lot of HIV in my system. This is due, in part, to me taking my medications and living a healthier life.

More important, I have gradually managed to come to terms with my HIV status. I've learned to forgive myself for being HIV positive. I don't consider this a punishment from God. I consider it sort of like a tap on the shoulder telling me that I need to take better care of myself and not be so reckless with my life.

Believe it or not, I also forgave the person who infected me. I had the opportunity to protect myself and I chose not to. I can live with that. Being angry at him or trying to be vengeful towards him will not make the HIV leave my body. I want to live a happy life, not a bitter one. Although he is no longer in my life, I know that I would be able to see him in the street and not want to get into a fistfight with him.

Now that I'm living with HIV I have learned to be grateful for what I have. The expensive medications I need are covered by my health insurance. There are so many in this world who don't even know they have HIV, or don't have access to the costly care they need.

I am looking forward to living a healthy, long life. My doctor tells me that if I take my medications and follow his orders, he can help me live to the age of 60. And with all the research going on about HIV, maybe, just maybe, they might come up with a cure.

The author was 23 when he wrote this story.
He graduated from college and got a job in media.

Why I Always Use a Condom

By Anonymous

It was raining outside and our plans were squashed. My girlfriend Kimberly and I had nothing to do. "Let's watch some TV," she said to me, but I had other plans. Little did I know they would lead to my biggest mistake.

We were alone in her house on that fall day five years ago. Her parents were at work. Sex wasn't anything new to us—we'd been steady lovers for almost a year. My plan was working to perfection when Kimberly stopped me.

"Do you have a condom?"

I told her I didn't.

"I don't want to have sex if you're not protected. You never know what could happen."

I told her not to worry, that it was no big deal if we didn't use a condom this one time. So we had sex. It was fun and made us both feel great.

But the pleasure we had that one afternoon couldn't compare with the pain that followed in the months to come. Kimberly didn't get her period. After a visit to the doctor, she found out she was pregnant.

She went crazy. She was crying, almost shaking. She talked about running away from home. When I told her that was a stupid idea, she began to scream that she was going to tell her mother.

I pleaded with Kimberly not to do that. We were only 14 and just starting high school. I didn't think telling our parents would help—it would only get us in more trouble and they would probably make us break up. Kimberly agreed not to tell as long as I made the arrangements and paid for the abortion.

It took two months to get the money together. Those two months were the worst of our lives. Kimberly was suffering emotionally and physically. She was depressed, vomiting, and had a headache every day. She had sudden mood swings and was growing quite distant. I was missing a lot of school and doing everything and anything to make money—odd jobs, gambling, robbing, stealing, lots of things I'm not proud of.

All I had to do, Kimberly said, was stay away and pretend I never knew her.

January came and, with it, the abortion date: January 3rd at 1:30 p.m. When I woke up that morning I was nervous and jittery. I just wanted the ordeal to end. We planned to meet at 1 p.m. at the doctor's office. At 2:30 I was still waiting. At 3 p.m. I finally called her house.

"Meet me down the block from my house," she said.

Now I knew there was trouble.

I got there in about a half-hour and asked her whe she had been.

"I felt sick."

I offered to get her an appointment the following day but she screamed "No!" She told me she woke up scared, couldn't take it any longer, and told her mother everything.

Her mother blamed me for what happened. "It's all his fault," she said. As horrible as it sounded when Kimberly told me this, her mother was right. It was my fault.

Then Kimberly's mother forbade her to have the abortion. I was off the hook—I didn't have to pay for it. All I had to do, Kimberly said, was stay away and pretend I never knew her. If I didn't, her mother threatened to tell my parents about the situation. I had no choice but to follow the rules.

As the weeks went by, I was dying to know how Kimberly was doing. Even though we weren't talking, I still loved her. I began to spy on her. I'd wait for her across the street from her house. I'd hide in the bushes or sit in a parked car. Sometimes I'd follow her and I began to notice that she was getting bigger. She was going to have a baby—my baby! I had to talk with her. When I saw her go out to the store one day, I stopped her.

"How are you?"

"Fine."

"Listen, you're having my baby. I think I should be a part of everything going on now.

"No, my mother and I agree you shouldn't be around. I don't want you around and I hate you!"

I could tell she wasn't really turning on me, just following her mother's orders. I was shocked and hurt, but there was nothing I could do.

Two months after the baby was born, they moved to Florida.

In the months that followed I lost all contact with her. It was May and school was nearly over. I should have been happy, but on the day vacation began I found out from a friend that Kimberly had gone into labor. I raced to the hospital.

"It's a boy!" I screamed in the hallway outside her room. I wanted to see my child, but her mother wouldn't allow me in. How could she do that? How could the hospital allow it? I argued, but it was no use.

I went to see Kimberly the night she got home from the hospital. Except for the hair and eyes, the baby looked exactly like me. I felt the joy of birth. Shortly afterwards her mother made me leave. On the way down to the bus I was jumped by three guys—friends of Kim's mom—who told me to leave Kimberly alone. "Stay away or we'll kill you!" they said.

I finally told my father everything. He was upset and disappointed, but he agreed to help me. After weeks of negotiations, Kimberly's mother agreed to visitation rights. Twice a month.

It was obvious, whenever I visited, that her mother was still angry.

Two months after the baby was born, they moved to Florida. They were gone for a month before I even found out.

I never stop thinking about what happened. And although I'll never give up responsibility for my son or be ashamed of him, I will always know that a mistake caused all this. We should have used a condom that day. Not only to protect ourselves, but to protect everyone around us who was affected by our behavior. My girlfriend became a mother at 14 and had to leave school. Her life was ruined and mine was changed forever. Had we been responsible that fall day five years ago, things might have worked out better.

In the last three years I've probably spent ten days with my son. I bounce him on my lap and play airplane with him, but he doesn't remember me and he doesn't call me Dad. I wonder, "Will he ever acknowledge me when I'm older? Will he ever understand?"

The author was in high school when he wrote this story.

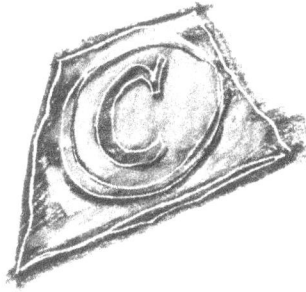

Practical Info

All About Birth Control, Right Here

By Rasheeda Raji and Kymberly Sheckleford

You must have heard it time and time again, but we're going to let you know one more time: abstinence, not having sex, is the only 100% sure method of avoiding pregnancy and sexually transmitted diseases (STDs), including HIV, the virus that causes AIDS. But if you do decide to have sex, protect yourself and your body by knowing how to get and use condoms.

On the next few pages, we've provided information on both the male and female condom, which are the only two contraceptives that can prevent STDs. We've also explained how the pill and other female birth control methods work. By using condoms and birth control together, you reduce two risks at once: the chance that you'll get an STD and the chance you'll have an unwanted pregnancy.

Because you are putting your body on the line for someone else, consider talking to your partner about birth control and condoms before you start messing around. Get familiar with one another's sexual history. Share your feelings and concerns about sexual activity. You want to make sure that you are making a decision that you won't regret later.

If you become sexually active, you're exposing yourself to a whole new range of possible medical conditions. It's more important than ever to maintain your health. If you're a woman, get regular gynecological (GYN) examinations and STD tests (see p. 302 for more on the GYN exam). If you're a man, get tested regularly for STDs.

Planned Parenthood offers confidential services to teens regardless of age or income, including GYN exams, all kinds of contraceptives, family planning counseling, emergency birth control, pregnancy testing, prenatal care, abortions, and HIV/STD testing. For the Planned Parenthood nearest you, call 1-800-230-PLAN or check www.plannedparenthood.org.

THE CONDOM

Description: A cover that fits over the penis and catches semen (cum) before, during, and after a man ejaculates (cums), preventing sperm from entering his partner's body. Condoms are usually made of latex. Some condoms, called "lambskin condoms," are made from animal tis-

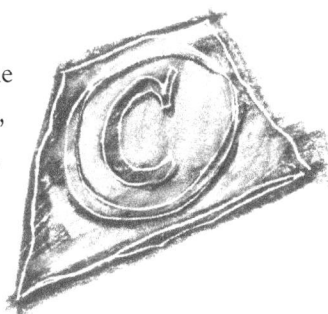

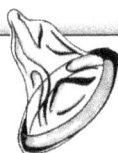

Condom Tips

• If a condom fails, both partners should wash their genitals with soap and water and urinate. Quickly applying a spermicide may also help. Girls should take emergency contraception (EC) as soon as possible (see p. 291 for more information).

• Even if you do it right, the condom can break. To avoid rips, use a water-based lubricant or a pre-lubricated condom. Do not use oil-based lubricants like lotion or petroleum jelly—they'll cause the condom to break.

• Extra-strength condoms are recommended for anal sex.

• Many condom packages print information about how to use a condom on the inside of the box. Open the package without too much ripping so you can carefully read the instructions and warnings.

• Condoms should be stored in a cool, dry place (not in wallets.) Heat, light, pressure, and air pollution can damage them.

sue. Lambskin condoms don't protect you from HIV and other STDs. Make sure the package says "latex condom." The condom is the only form of birth control that men can use to prevent pregnancy. The condom and the female condom are the only birth control methods that protect against STDs.

Effectiveness: Of 100 women whose partners use condoms when they have sex, about 15 will become pregnant during the first year of typical use. Typical use rates take into account that most people won't use condoms correctly every time. Using condoms correctly includes putting one on before you start rubbing up against each other naked (because

How to Use a Male Condom
(as demonstrated on a banana)

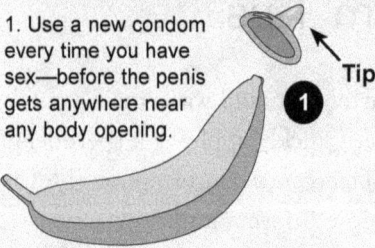

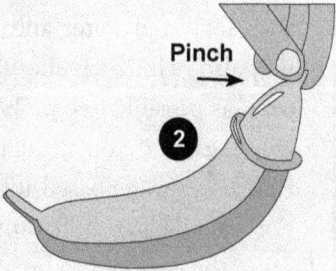

1. Use a new condom every time you have sex—before the penis gets anywhere near any body opening.

Tip

Pinch

Women can get pregnant from pre-ejaculate fluid (pre-cum), and both men and women can get STDs from skin-to-skin contact. Check the condom's expiration date and open the package carefully, since teeth or fingernails can tear the latex. Put the condom on as soon as the penis gets hard. If the penis is uncircumsized, pull back foreskin.

2. Make sure the rolled-up ring is on the outside. Handling the condom gently, pinch the tip so no air is trapped inside, and allow room for semen if you come.

semen can leak out of the penis before a man cums). It also means being careful about how you put the condom on and take it off. Being careful is worth it: Only 2 in every 100 women will become pregnant if condoms are used perfectly.

Because condoms help protect against HIV and other infections, anyone who is having vaginal (penis in vagina) or anal (penis in anus) intercourse should use them. To protect against STDs, you should also use a condom during oral (penis in mouth) sex.

Because it can break or slip off if not used correctly, the condom is more effective as birth control when used with spermicide, which is a sperm-killing foam, film, cream, insert, or jelly. Some condoms come

3. Hold the tip while you unroll the condom all the way to the base of the penis.
   If it doesn't unroll, it's on backwards. Throw the condom away and start over with a new one.
   Make sure that it fits and isn't loose. Experiment with different brands to get the right size.

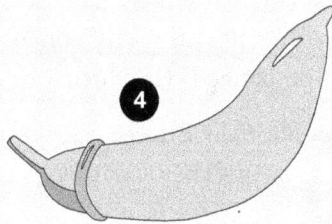

4. You're ready.

3 Unroll

5 Hold base

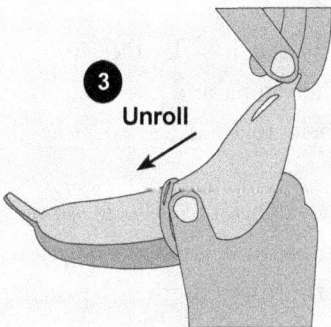

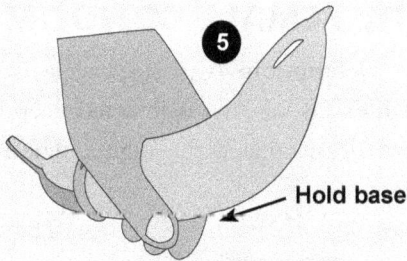

5. After sex: Pull out slowly while you're still hard. Hold the base of the condom to avoid spilling semen.
   Dispose of it properly. Don't flush it down the toilet.

with spermicide already inside them; the label will say "spermicidal lubricant."

Pros: Condoms help prevent the spread of HIV and other STDs. They are inexpensive and easy to get. You can buy them at any drugstore without a prescription, and many clinics and some high schools make them available for free. Since condoms are small and lightweight, it's easy to carry them with you at all times. They make it possible for men to take responsibility for birth control. They may also help a man stay erect longer.

Cons: You have to use one every time you have intercourse. Putting the condom on may feel awkward or uncomfortable at first since it must be used right at the time of intercourse. It may also dull sensation for either partner. It may tear or come off during intercourse, especially if it's not put on correctly (see directions on pp. 282-283).

Possible Side Effects: There are none, except for people who are allergic to latex. (They can use plastic condoms, which are just as effective as latex.)

Cost: Condoms cost $7–$13 per dozen at drugstores and supermarkets. Many clinics give them out for free.

THE FEMALE CONDOM

Description: A plastic baggie-like pouch that has flexible rings on each end. One ring is inserted deep into the vagina and the other ring stays open outside the vagina. The rings help to hold the condom in place.

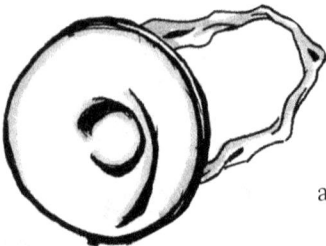

The female condom collects semen before, during, and after ejaculation, keeping sperm from entering the vagina and protecting against pregnancy and STDs. Female condoms should not be used at the same time as male condoms.

Insertion of Female Condom

Uterus

Cervix

Inner ring
of condom

Vagina

Outer ring
of condom

For more detailed instructions,
read the condom's package.

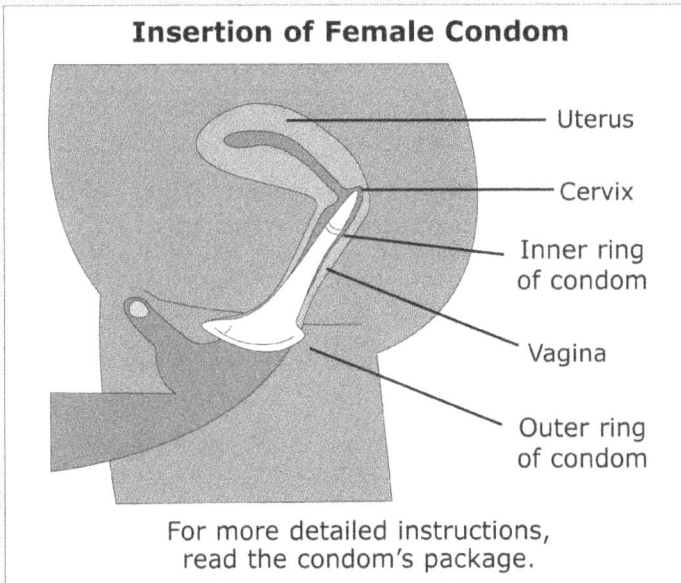

Effectiveness: With typical use, 21 out of every 100 women using female condoms will get pregnant in a year. With perfect use, 5 out of 100 will get pregnant. Spermicide increases effectiveness.

Pros: The female condom helps prevent many STDs (including HIV and AIDS), and can be used for both anal and vaginal sex. The female condom can be purchased at a drugstore without a prescription. It allows women to take responsibility for STD prevention without having to rely on their partners. And it can be used by people who are allergic to latex.

Cons: Female condoms can be tricky to use. They can only be used once. They are generally more expensive than male condoms.

Possible Side Effects: May cause irritation.

Price: You can pick up free female condoms at some clinics and other organizations. At a drugstore, a pack of three female condoms is about $17.

HORMONAL CONTRACEPTIVES

The pill, the patch, the ring, Depo-Provera, and Implanon are all forms of birth control that work by releasing hormones that prevent your body from producing eggs. When used correctly, they are very effective at preventing pregnancy. However, **none of these methods protect against HIV and other STDs.** To protect yourself from infection, you must also use a condom.

THE PILL

Description: A monthly series of pills—you take one birth control tablet a day. Basically, the pill has hormones that prevent pregnancy by stopping the release of eggs from your ovaries.

Effectiveness: With typical use, 8 women out of 100 will get pregnant while taking the pill. With perfect use (taking it every day at the same time), fewer than 1 out of 100 women will become pregnant. However, it may take a week or two for the pill to become effective.

Pros: The pill is good for women who are disciplined (because you have to remember to take it at the same time every day—missing a pill can lead to pregnancy). Women who use the pill have more regular periods, less menstrual flow, less cramping, less iron deficiency and anemia, less pelvic inflammatory disease (PID), and less premenstrual tension than women who don't take it. Also, it can reduce acne.

Cons: The pill doesn't protect against HIV or other STDs. You need a doctor's prescription to get the pill. You must take it every day at the same time, even when you aren't planning to have sex. Women who take it may be at slightly greater risk for some medical conditions like blood clots, heart attack, and stroke—ask your doctor about this. Smoking increases your risk for some of these conditions, so doctors recommend

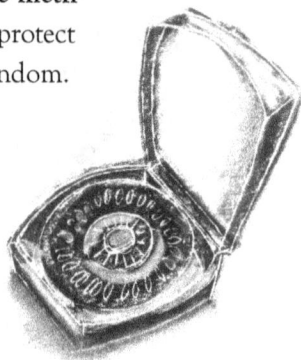

that you do not smoke when you are on the pill.

Possible Side Effects: Many women don't have any side effects, and for those who do, most side effects go away after two or three months. The pill can cause nausea, vomiting, headaches, mood changes, weight gain or loss, breast tenderness, or bleeding between periods.

Price: The pill costs anywhere from $10-50 a month, depending on what kind you take, whether or not it's covered by your insurance, and whether you buy it at a drugstore or a clinic. (Clinics are usually cheaper and sometimes offer a reduced rate based on income.) You must have a prescription.

There are several other, less popular kinds of hormonal contraceptive methods, including the patch, the ring, Depo-Provera, and Implanon. Like the pill, none of these methods prevent sexually transmitted infections, but they are highly effective in preventing pregnancy. All the hormonal contraceptives require a prescription. A brief overview of each:

THE PATCH

The patch is a thin piece of plastic that is worn on the buttocks, stomach, upper arm, or upper torso (but never on the breasts). Use one patch per week for three weeks in a row. On the fourth week, you don't wear a patch and you get your period. Side effects are similar to the pill. It's about $15-50 per month.

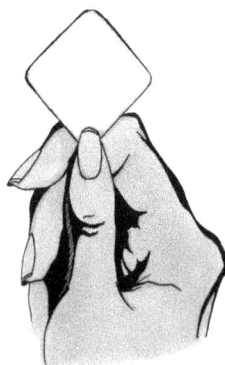

THE RING

The ring is a soft and flexible plastic ring that's inserted into the vagina. Only one ring is needed for three weeks of use, though you must remember to remove it exactly 21 days after you put it in, and replace it

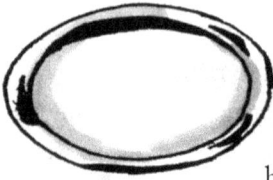

one week after that. Inserting the ring may be awkward at first. Side effects may include mood swings, headache, nausea, vaginal discharge, breast tenderness, weight gain or loss, bleeding between periods, and vaginal irritation. It is also about $15–50 a month.

With typical use 8 women out of 100 will get pregnant while using the ring or the patch. With perfect use, fewer than 1 out of 100 women will become pregnant.

DEPO-PROVERA

Depo-Provera is a shot that you get injected into your body every 11-13 weeks with a needle. That means, you only have to worry about birth control four times a year. However, if you don't like it and want to stop using it, you'll have to suffer through any side effects you've been experiencing for up to three months while waiting for your last injection to wear off. Irregular periods are common. Less common side effects may include increased appetite and weight gain, headache, sore breasts, nausea, nervousness, dizziness, depression, skin rashes or spotty darkening of the skin, hair loss, increased hair on face or body, and increased or decreased sex drive.

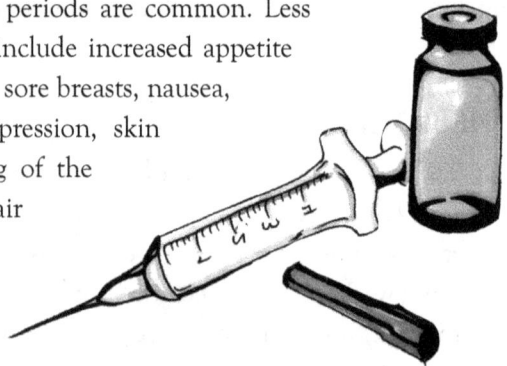

The initial doctor's visit to get Depo-Provera can be $35–250 and injections are $35–75 four times a year. You may have to pay exam fees between $20–40 during each visit, as well. You should not use it continuously for more than two years.

IMPLANON

Another highly effective hormonal birth control method is Implanon, or implantable contraception. Implanon is a small, matchstick-sized flexible plastic tube containing hormones that doctors insert just under the skin of the upper arm. It protects against pregnancy for up to three years. However, it's expensive. The cost of the exam, Implanon, and insertion ranges from $400–800. Removal costs between $75 and $150. Medicaid and private health insurance may cover it. Possible side effects are similar to the pill, plus irritation, infection, and possible scarring where the tubes are inserted.

Both Depo-Provera and Implanon are convenient and highly effective—fewer than 1 out of 100 women who use either correctly will get pregnant.

BARRIER METHOD CONTRACEPTIVES

Like condoms, the diaphragm and cervical cap help prevent pregnancy by blocking sperm from entering the uterus. However, **neither of these methods protect against HIV and other STDs**. To protect yourself from infection, you must also use a condom.

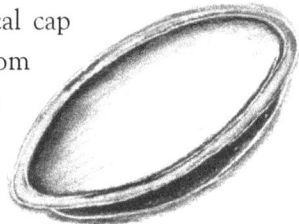

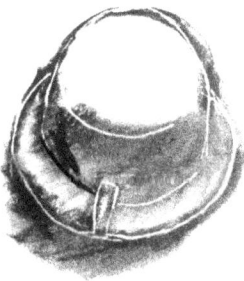

The **diaphragm** is a soft silicone or latex cup that you fill with spermicide and insert into the vagina up to six hours before sex. A **cervical cap** is similar to a diaphragm, but smaller, and can be inserted up to 40 hours before sex. You must see a doctor and get fitted to get one. There are almost no side effects or health risks for either of these methods, but they are less effective than hormonal birth control: Out of 100 women who use them, 14–16 will become pregnant during the first year of typical use.

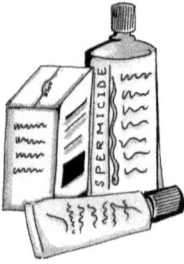

Both barrier methods must be used with **spermicide**, a sperm-killing chemical that can be bought at drugstores. (Spermicides come in many forms, including film, inserts, foam, cream, and jelly, and cost about $8–18 per tube. A tube will last a while.)

Rasheeda was 20 and Kymberly was 17 when they wrote this story. Rasheeda went on to earn an undergraduate degree from the University of Virginia and a law degree from Howard University; Kymberly graduated from the State University of New York at Purchase.

All About Emergency Contraception

If a condom breaks or you have unprotected sex, it's still possible to protect yourself from getting pregnant by taking the "morning after pill," also known as emergency contraception (EC) or Plan B. Emergency contraceptives do not protect you from STDs (sexually transmitted diseases).

You can use emergency contraception up to five days after having unprotected sex. However, it is most effective if taken within 72 hours (three days) after having unprotected sex. The sooner you take these pills, the more likely they'll prevent pregnancy. Emergency contraception pills work in a few ways. They can stop an egg and sperm from meeting, or stop the egg from attaching to the uterus so you can't get pregnant.

Short-term side effects may include nausea, fatigue, and breast tenderness. Your menstrual period may be temporarily irregular after taking EC.

Emergency contraception is safe, but it shouldn't be used in place of birth control because it's not healthy to take it often and it's not as effective as many other kinds of birth control. Even if you take it within three days, it prevents pregnancy only 75-89% of the time.

The cost of emergency contraception varies a great deal, depending on where you go and what services you need. Plan B may cost $35-55, but many local health departments offer EC for free or at a reduced cost for low-income women.

If you're 17 or older, you can get EC at your local pharmacy or health clinic without a prescription. If you're under 17, you must first get a prescription for EC from a clinic or your doctor's office, or you can ask a friend or family member who is 17 or older to buy EC for you at a pharmacy.

To find a list of locations that provide emergency contraception,

call: **(1-888) NOT-2-LATE (1-888-668-2528)**

or visit: **http://ECLocator.not-2-late.com**

If you have other questions about pregnancy, or want to find a Planned Parenthood health center, go to www.plannedparenthood.org or call 1-800-230-PLAN.

All About STDs

The last thing you want to do when you're having sex is get a disease, or give one to your partner. Sexually transmitted diseases (STDs) are very serious, but you can take steps to protect yourself and your partner. Here's what you need to know:

Who gets STDs?

The fact is that teens and young adults are most likely to be infected. There are about 19 million new STD infections each year, almost half of them among people ages 15 to 24. A recent study estimated that 1 in every 4 teen girls has been infected with at least one of the four most common STDs (chlamydia, genital herpes, HPV and trichomoniasis).

How do you get an STD?

STDs are primarily spread through sexual contact such as vaginal sex (penis to vagina) anal sex (penis to anus) or oral sex (penis, vagina, or anus to mouth). If you are having sex, you are at risk of getting an STD, regardless of whether you are having sex with women, men, or both.

How can you prevent STDs?

The only completely sure way is to practice abstinence (don't have sex). If you are sexually active, using a barrier method, like a condom every time you have sex, including oral sex, will reduce your risk.

How do you treat an STD?

Trichomoniasis, chlamydia, gonorrhea and syphilis can be cured with antibiotics. Be careful—after being cured, you can still get re-infected.

Herpes and HIV (the virus that causes AIDS) have no cure—they stay in your body for life. But medication can help reduce the symptoms.

There is no treatment for HPV, but it can be prevented with a new vaccine, which can protect you against the strain of HPV that causes cervical cancer. It's best if you get the vaccine before becoming sexually active.

Who should get tested?

If you've ever had sex, you should get tested for HIV and other STDs. Even if you've had protected sex, you should still get tested, since no method is 100% effective. You can often get tested for free, and don't need a parent or guardian's permission. For more information on how to get tested, talk to your doctor or go to www.hivtest.org.

COMMON STDS AND HOW TO TREAT THEM

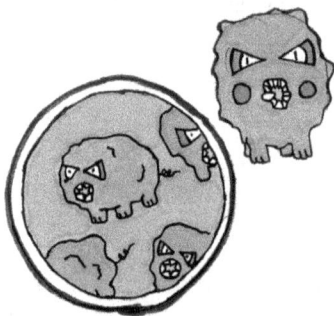

HIV/AIDS

What It Is: HIV stands for human immunodeficiency virus. This is the virus that causes AIDS. HIV attacks the immune system, the body system that helps us fight infections. When HIV weakens the immune system to a certain level, then the person has AIDS, a disease in which the body can no longer fight off infections. Ultimately, the disease causes death.

About 1 million people in the United States are living with HIV or AIDS. About a quarter don't know that they are infected. Not knowing puts them and others at risk. Each year more than 56,000 people get infected with HIV.

Symptoms: The only way to know whether you are infected is to get tested regularly for HIV. Someone can look and feel healthy but can still be infected; it can take years for symptoms to show up.

How You Catch HIV: HIV lives in the blood, semen (cum) or vaginal fluid of an infected person. HIV is transmitted in two main ways: (1) Having anal, vaginal, or oral sex with someone infected with HIV; (2) sharing needles and syringes with someone infected with HIV. (Infected mothers can pass the virus on to their children during pregnancy or through breast feeding. People can also get HIV through blood transfusions, though that's very rare now).

How to Prevent HIV: Always use a latex condom for vaginal, anal and oral sex. Get tested and talk to your sex partner about getting tested. If you are infected, tell your current and former partners. And if you are taking intravenous drugs (shooting up) never share needles.

How to Treat HIV: There is no cure. But there are now drugs that let many HIV-positive people live longer, healthier lives. These drugs help control the outbreak of the virus, but they have a lot of side effects that can impact your quality of life, such as causing chronic diarrhea.

GENITAL HERPES

What It Is: Genital herpes is caused by the herpes simplex virus (HSV). There are two kinds: Type 1 (oral herpes, cold sores on the mouth) or Type 2 (genital herpes).

Nationwide, at least 45 million people ages 12 and older, or one out of five people, have had genital HSV infection.

Symptoms: Blisters on or near the genitals (penis or vagina) or rectum. These sores may take two to four weeks to heal the first time they occur. You may also have flu-like symptoms, including fever and swollen glands. Another "outbreak" of sores can appear weeks or months after the first. These outbreaks are usually shorter and less painful. A person can have about four to five outbreaks a year.

However, many people have no symptoms—

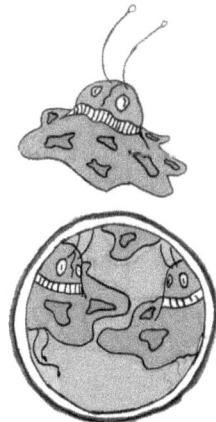

and they still can infect others. Usually people are only contagious while they're having an outbreak, but an outbreak can begin before you notice it.

How You Catch Herpes: Most genital herpes is caused by HSV-2, which spreads through contact with the infected area—usually vaginal or anal sex. HSV-1 can be transmitted to the genitals through oral sex.

How to Prevent Herpes: Use latex condoms for genital, anal and oral sex. Get tested and if you are infected, tell your current and former sex partners. Do not have sex during an outbreak.

Genital HSV can lead to deadly infections in babies. It is especially important for women to get tested for herpes when they know they're pregnant, and avoid getting herpes during pregnancy (by avoiding unprotected sex). If you know you have herpes and are pregnant, make sure to tell your doctor immediately.

How to Treat Herpes: There is no cure; you have herpes for life. Doctors are working on a herpes vaccine, and there are antiviral drugs to reduce the number and intensity of outbreaks.

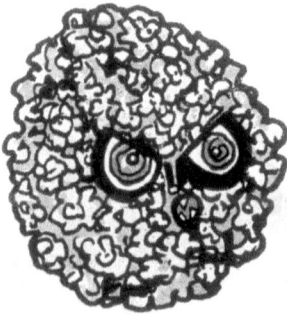

HPV

What It Is: Genital human papillomavirus (HPV) infects the skin and mucous membranes. There are more than 40 HPV types that can infect the genital areas, including the penis, vulva (area outside the vagina), and anus, and the linings of the vagina, cervix and rectum.

HPV is the most common sexually transmitted infection. At least half of sexually active men and women get a genital HPV infection at some point in their lives.

Symptoms: Most people with HPV don't get symptoms or health problems. But certain types can cause genital warts in men and women one to six months after they catch it. Other HPV types can cause cervical cancer and other less common cancers, such as cancers of the vulva, vagina, anus and penis. The types of HPV that cause genital warts are not the same as the types that can cause cancer.

Genital warts usually appear as small bumps usually in the genital area. They can appear on the vulva, in or around the vagina or anus, on the cervix, and on the penis, scrotum, groin, or thigh. Warts may appear within weeks or months after sexual contact with an infected person—or they may not appear at all.

How You Catch HPV: Skin-to-skin contact with warts—but those warts could be hidden inside the urethra (urine canal) or vaginal walls.

How to Prevent HPV: A new vaccine can now protect females from the four types of HPV that cause most cervical cancers and genital warts. It is given in three doses, which should be started before girls become sexually active. The vaccine will not protect you if you've already been infected with HPV. Using a condom will also reduce the risk of infection.

How to Treat HPV: HPV often goes away on its own, without causing health problems. But there's no guarantee. Most people who become infected with HPV do not even know they have it. You should get tested for signs of disease that HPV can cause, especially cervical cancer.

TRICHOMONIASIS

What It Is: Trichomoniasis is caused by a tiny parasite. The vagina is where women are usually infected. The urethra (urine canal) is the most common site of infection in men.

Trichomoniasis is the most common curable STD in young, sexually active women.

Symptoms: Symptoms are more common in women and usually appear within five to 28 days of exposure. Symptoms include yellowish green vaginal discharge with a strong odor; itching; pain during urination and/or intercourse; and urinary tract infections. Most men with trichomoniasis do not have signs or symptoms; however, some men may

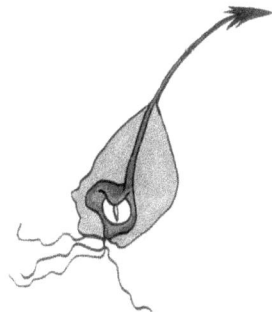

temporarily have an irritation inside the penis, mild discharge, or slight burning after urination or ejaculation.

How You Catch Trichomoniasis: The parasite is spread through penis-to-vagina intercourse or vulva-to-vulva contact with an infected partner. Women can catch the disease from infected men or women, but men usually contract it only from infected women.

How to Prevent Trichomoniasis: Condoms and dental dams can help prevent it. Stop having sex if you have any of the above symptoms— and get tested.

How to Treat Trichomoniasis: Antibiotics, usually taken in one dose, will get rid of it. Your sexual partner/s should get treated at the same time so they don't re-infect you.

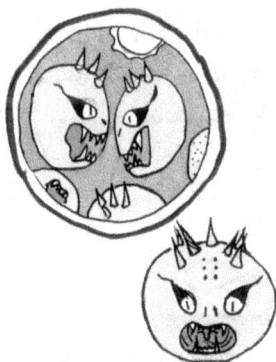

CHLAMYDIA

What It Is: Chlamydia is a bacterial infection that can lead to serious reproductive problems for women.

Chlamydia is the most common infectious disease in the U.S.: Over one million cases are reported a year. Many more cases go undiagnosed—as many as 2.8 million new cases each year.

Symptoms: Most women never have symptoms, so you should get tested every year. Women who do get symptoms may have abnormal vaginal discharge, painful urination, fever, nausea, or pain during sex. Men may have discharge from the penis, burning or itching in the urethra or pain or swelling in the testicles.

How You Catch Chlamydia: Genital-to-genital and genital-to-anal contact.

How to Prevent Chlamydia: Sex with a condom can help prevent chlamydia.

How to Treat Chlamydia: It can easily be cured with antibiotics, which can clear up the infection in about 7-10 days. If you find out you have it, your partner should get tested and treated as well, so you don't get re-infected.

If left untreated, chlamydia can cause severe health consequences for women, including pelvic inflammatory disease (PID). PID is an infection of the uterus, fallopian tubes and/or ovaries that can lead to ectopic pregnancy and infertility. Up to 40 percent of females with untreated chlamydia infections develop PID, and 20 percent of those may become infertile.

GONORRHEA

What It Is: A bacterial infection that enters the body through mucous membranes in the vagina, urethra, cervix, anus and mouth.

Gonorrhea is the second most commonly reported infectious disease in the U.S.

Symptoms: Most people don't have symptoms. Those who do may have abnormal discharge from vagina or penis and pain during urination.

How You Catch Gonorrhea: Genital, oral or anal sex.

How to Prevent Gonorrhea: Using a condom during sex helps reduce the risk, but again, is not 100% effective.

How to Treat Gonorrhea: Antibiotics can get rid of it, but a growing number of gonorrhea cases are resistant to the antibiotic that has been used to treat it.

You should get tested for gonorrhea and chlamydia at the same time, since they often occur together, and neither shows symptoms. If left untreated, gonorrhea in men can cause epididymitis, a painful infection in the tissue around the testicles that can lead to infertility. Like chlamydia, untreated gonorrhea in women can lead to Pelvic Inflammatory Disease, which can make it difficult to get pregnant and also cause infertility.

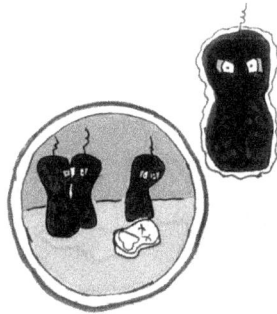

SYPHILIS

What It Is: Syphilis is a disease caused by bacteria that enter the body through the mucous membranes or cuts in the skin.

Six times more men than women have syphilis, partly due to its prevalence among men who have sex with men.

Symptoms: If untreated, syphilis develops in four stages.

First Stage: Painless, red-rimmed sores on genitals, anus or mouth. These can last for about three to six weeks.

Second Stage: This happens six weeks to six months later. Symptoms include a rash all over the body or on the palms and bottoms of feet, and bad flu-like symptoms like fever and nausea as well as joint swelling and hair loss. This lasts one to eight weeks.

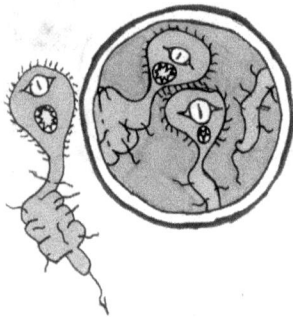

Third Stage: If syphilis is not treated in the first two stages, it can "hide" for years. You won't have any symptoms, but the disease is still in your body.

Fourth Stage: This happens 10-20 years later. At this point, the infection has spread throughout your body and can cause brain damage, heart disease, paralysis and even death.

How You Catch Syphilis: Syphilis is spread by contact with the sores or through genital-to-genital, genital-to-oral, or genital-to-anal contact. Like many other STDs, it can help spread HIV, because the HIV virus can easily enter the sores during unprotected sex.

How to Prevent Syphilis: Using a condom can help. It's especially important for pregnant women not to have or get syphilis: It can cause physical deformity and brain and nervous system complications in children, stillbirth and death soon after birth.

How to Treat Syphilis: Antibiotics can cure syphilis in its early stages. However, the longer the infection remains in your system, the more treatment is required. It's important to get tested and treated as soon as possible.

GETTING TESTED

It can be scary to acknowledge that you might have an STD. But if you've had unprotected sex, you need to get tested. Many STDs can be easily cured. And the ones that can't, like herpes and HIV, can be controlled. For your own health—and that of your partner—you need to know if you have anything. Private doctors, city health departments, and many other clinics offer testing, and it's often free and confidential. For more information and to find a testing center near you, go to ww.hivtest.org or plannedparenthood.org, or talk to your doctor.

The GYN Exam, Explained

By Madeleine Gordillo

"OK, you're all done," the nurse-practitioner told me to my surprise. I didn't say anything but I was thinking, "You mean, that's it?!" I was expecting my first gynecological exam to last a lifetime. It ended up taking a whole seven minutes.

When I first started thinking about getting this exam, I was nervous. I pictured it being a horrible experience, because the few times I'd heard girls talk about it they would say things like, "They stick a metal thing in you, open you up, and poke at you." I don't take pain very well and I wasn't comfortable with the idea of having a stranger examine me that intimately, so I wasn't too excited about getting the exam.

I was also hesitant because I didn't want to deal with the doctor or nurse asking me questions about my private life that I would feel uncomfortable answering. And I was concerned about what my family and friends would think of me. I knew I would be getting questions like, "What've you been doing that you need to get a test?" or "What's wrong with you, are you sick?" I worried that they would get the wrong idea. I wasn't thinking about getting the exam because I thought I was pregnant or had an STD—I knew that wasn't the case. I just wanted to learn more about my body.

There is a lot of information that women, especially teenagers, must know about their constantly changing bodies. Once you start menstruating, you may have symptoms related to your period and the hormones your body starts producing. I decided the GYN exam was something girls needed to do to take care of our health and that I would be losing out if I didn't get one.

I read up on the examination and asked questions but I still had concerns about things like where to have it done. I wanted to go to a doctor or clinic that would be gentle in all ways. I felt I needed people who were going to take the time out to talk to me and prepare me for what was to come. I also knew I wanted an extremely sanitary place — if they weren't careful with how they cared for their workplace, I knew they wouldn't be careful with me.

I had heard that Planned Parenthood offered free services for young people in high school, including GYN exams. I decided to call them and ask for a tour of their clinic to see what I would be getting myself into. The tour of the clinic eased my anxiety a lot because I was able to see where I would be seen and what I would be examined with. I found out that I would get to speak to a counselor before the exam and I was also shown a detailed video of a real GYN exam which explained what they would be doing and the reasons for it. (The purpose of the exam is to check for any signs of infection or disease, like irregular lumps in the breasts, redness and/or inflammation of the vagina, unusual vaginal discharges, etc.) After taking the clinic tour, watching the video and talking to a few people, I was confident that I wanted to go ahead and have the exam.

Getting a GYN exam is probably one of the best things a girl can do for herself.

The day of the exam, I must admit there were still butterflies in my stomach. I expected it to be painful but all I felt was slight pressure at some points. I worried that I might not feel comfortable talking to the counselor, but in reality she turned out to be one of the most welcoming and understanding people I'd ever met. In regards to my family and friends' reactions, they were stunned but ultimately proud of me, as I was of myself. In the end, none of my fears turned out to be justified.

I learned a lot of invaluable things about my body and character that day. For example, I am now able to differentiate between a normal lump on my breast and one that I should consult with a doctor about. More importantly than that, I learned how important it is to become comfortable checking your own body and to care enough about yourself to do so. Now, as I talk from experience, I can sincerely tell you that getting a GYN exam is probably one of the best things a girl can do for herself.

Here's what the exam was like, step-by-step:

Your visit to the gynecologist begins like any doctor's appointment—you fill out forms about your medical history and your reasons for being there.

Next, you may be asked for blood and urine samples for pregnancy testing. At some clinics, you will then get to speak to a counselor before getting examined by a doctor or nurse-practitioner. She'll go over the information you revealed on the forms and confirm some of the details. (For example, if you wrote that there is diabetes in your family, she'll ask which family member has it.) Then the counselor will ask you why you are there. If you came for something specific, like to get birth control, you should tell her that.

She will also answer any questions you might have about the exam, and try to address any concerns or fears you might have about it, especially if it's your first time. The counselor will ask you such things as whose idea it was that you have the exam (they want to be sure you're not being pressured into it by anyone, like your mother or a boyfriend), if you are sexually active, whether you use protection when you have sex, and so on.

After the counseling session, you are directed to the examining room. You are asked to take off your clothes and change into a paper robe. Then you'll be asked to sit on an examining table with small metal hoops, called stirrups, attached to the bottom corners. They keep your legs spread apart so that the doctor will be able to examine you properly. When the doctor comes in, she'll direct you to lie on the bed with the heels of your feet in the stirrups.

The examination begins with a breast exam. The doctor will open your robe and tell you to place both hands behind your head. Using the flat side of her three middle fingers, she'll feel for any abnormal lumps in your breasts and armpits. The doctor will also teach you how to examine your own breasts between doctors' visits.

Next comes the pelvic exam. First, the doctor will check the outer surface of your vagina to make sure everything looks normal. Then comes the scary part—inserting the speculum. This is the instrument used to hold the walls of the vagina open so the doctor can see inside. These instruments are "L" shaped. One side is the handle the doctor holds. The other side, the part that goes inside you, reminds me of the bill of a pelican since it is a long and narrow and opens and closes like a mouth.

While it is in its closed position, the doctor will gently insert the speculum into your vagina. Once it's in place, she will open the mouth of the speculum. Many people fear that this will be painful, but if you relax and don't tense up, all you should feel is a slight pressure. The doctor will check the walls of your vagina and the opening of your cervix for any abnormalities (redness, inflammation, cysts, unusual discharge) that could be signs of infection or disease. If you have any questions about your reproductive organs or about what the doctor is doing, you should feel free to ask them during the exam.

Next, the doctor will insert a longer than average version of a Q-tip into your vagina to get some cell samples (you might feel some "poking" at this point). This is called the Pap smear and it is done to test for warning signs of cancer. If you are sexually active, the doctor may take another sample to test you for gonorrhea and chlamydia (both are STDs). This lasts about a minute. Then the doctor closes the speculum and eases it out.

Next she changes her gloves and spreads some KY jelly (a lubricant) on one or two of her fingers. That's because, in order to examine your internal organs, she needs to place her finger(s) inside your vagina so she can feel your cervix. You will feel a little pressure at this point. With her other hand, the doctor will press down on your lower abdomen to feel your uterus and ovaries. She does this to feel for any abnormal swelling, tenderness or lumps.

That completes the exam. The doctor will probably spend a few minutes discussing it with you when you're done. You will be told if anything abnormal was found during the exam, such as inflammation of the vagina, any unusual lumps and/or unusual discharge. The doctor might prescribe something for it or tell you that you need additional tests. If you are sexually active, you should ask the doctor about taking an HIV test.

It usually takes a few days for the doctor to get the results of your Pap smear and STD culture. If anything irregular shows up in those test results, she'll contact you. If you don't hear from her, and you weren't told to call for the results, then everything's fine. To stay healthy, doctors recommend that you have a GYN exam once a year.

---

*Madeleine was 17 when she wrote this story. She graduated
high school and studied International Relations at Syracuse University.*

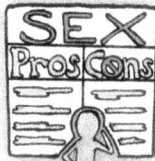

Are You Ready?

Still wondering if you're ready to have sex? Take this quiz with your partner, then turn the page to figure out your score.

1. Do you know why you want to have sex?
    ☐ Yes   ☐ No

2. Do you know which gender you're attracted to?
    ☐ Yes   ☐ No

3. Have you masturbated?
    ☐ Yes   ☐ No

4. Have you gone as far as you can go before having sex?
    ☐ Yes   ☐ No

5. Do you feel attractive?
    ☐ Yes   ☐ No

6. Do you know who you want to do it with?
    ☐ Yes   ☐ No

7. Does this person know how you really feel about him (or her)?
    ☐ Yes   ☐ No

8. Do you know how this person really feels about you?
    ☐ Yes   ☐ No

9. Does this person really care about you and make you feel special?
    ☐ Yes   ☐ No

10. Do you know their favorite color?
    ☐ Yes   ☐ No

11. What they're afraid of?
    ☐ Yes   ☐ No

12. The names of their brothers and sisters and best friends?
      ☐ Yes   ☐ No

13. Do you *really* like to kiss this person?
      ☐ Yes   ☐ No

14. Do you like the way this person smells?
      ☐ Yes   ☐ No

15. Has this person seen you on a bad hair day, and vice versa?
      ☐ Yes   ☐ No

16 Are you willing to have him or her see you walk around naked, with the lights on?
      ☐ Yes   ☐ No

17. Would you be able to handle it if this person broke up with you after having sex?
      ☐ Yes   ☐ No

18. Are you pretty close to the same age?
      ☐ Yes   ☐ No

19. Can you have a real and honest conversation with this person?
      ☐ Yes   ☐ No

20. Have you said "no" when you didn't want to do something?
      ☐ Yes   ☐ No

21. Have you talked about what kind of contraception you would use?
      ☐ Yes   ☐ No

22. Have you talked about how you would handle pregnancy or an STD?
      ☐ Yes   ☐ No

23. Do you feel safe with this person?
      ☐ Yes   ☐ No

24. Have you imagined how you'll feel afterwards?
      ☐ Yes   ☐ No

To score the quiz:

• Give yourself one point for each "Yes" answer.

• Give yourself 10 extra points if you've compared your answers with your partner's and talked about them.

• Then turn to p. 315 to see what your score means.

RESOURCES

Teen Sexuality Websites

www.plannedparenthood.org/teen-talk

The teen section of Planned Parenthood's website is informative and easy to understand. It includes fun videos and animation (on subjects like "How Pregnancy Happens") as well as articles and Q&As covering physical and mental health, relationships, and sexuality.

www.goaskalice.columbia.edu

Run by the Columbia University Health Service, this site provides straightforward, non-judgmental, sometimes humorous answers to your questions about sex, health, and relationships. It includes an archive of hundreds of Q&As organized by topic and continues to post new Q&As all the time. At "Go Ask Alice," there is truly no such thing as a dumb or embarrassing question. Some queries asked and answered on the site have been: "What happens to semen after it has been ejaculated into a woman's body?" "Is giving oral sex dangerous if you wear braces?" and "Help! I can't find my girlfriend's clitoris."

www.sexetc.org

Sex, etc. features accessible, teen-written articles on sex and relationships. The site also includes videos, comics and quizzes, answers to frequently asked questions, and forums where you can respond to other users and get your own questions answered. Sponsored by the Rutgers University Center for Family Life Education.

www.scarleteen.com

A fun, frank, informative site with great articles on topics like "First Intercourse 101" (what to expect your first time), "Shown Actual Size: A Penis Shape and Size Lowdown," and "Ready or Not" (a series of well-thought out checklists to help you figure out whether you're ready to have sex), along with advice columns, topical bulletin boards, and resource listings.

www.youthresource.com

A website by and for LGBTQ young people, created by Advocates for Youth, an organization that works to improve sexual health education and services for teens. This site features tons of information on health, advocacy, and "Queer Living," including great articles by young people on topics like growing up gay in rural areas and negotiating faith and spirituality issues. In the "Peer Support" section you can read about the peer educators who contribute to the site, and send in your questions.

Resources for Survivors of Sexual Abuse and Relationship Abuse

Rape, Abuse, and Incest National Network (RAINN)
www.rainn.org
1-800-656-HOPE

Free and confidential crisis support, answers to your questions, and referrals to other sources of help near you. You can call their 24-hour hotline or use the online version on their website (you chat with a trained volunteer through a private IM session). The website also contains lots of useful information about sexual assault, including how to protect yourself and how to recover.

National Teen Dating Abuse Helpline
www.loveisrespect.org
1-866-331-9474

If you're worried that you or a friend may be involved in an abusive relationship, call their 24-hour helpline or go to the website to chat with a trained peer advocate. The website also includes quizzes, tip sheets and articles about healthy and unhealthy relationships and the warning signs of abuse.

Books

Changing Bodies, Changing Lives, by Ruth Bell, et. al.
Published by Three Rivers Press

A great source for all the standard sex ed info about your body, how it works, and the kind of changes you can expect during adolescence, complete with illustrations. And there's more. As the title suggests, this book isn't just about sexuality but about the whole process of growing up and how it affects your sense of self and your relationships with your family, friends, boyfriends and girlfriends. One thing that sets *Changing Bodies* apart from other books covering the same topics is that it is full of teen voices — the experiences and observations of real teens are used to explain and illustrate the physical and emotional changes people go through during the junior high and high school years.

The Go Ask Alice Book of Answers: A Guide to Good Physical, Sexual, and Emotional Health, by Columbia University's Health Education Program. Published by Henry Holt and Company.

A collection of Q&As from the website (see p. 311), covers a wide range of physical and emotional issues, from how to kiss to how to know whether you've had an orgasm to how to cope with being dumped. The book also includes helpful advice on topics not directly related to sex like coping with depression, recovering from a hangover, and becoming a vegetarian.

The Sex Book: An Alphabet of Smarter Love, by Jane Pavanel.
Published by Lobster Press (Canada).

This informative, chatty book follows an A to Z format, providing definitions of terms like "cunnilingus," "chancroid" and "smegma" as well discussions of harder to pin down concepts like "masculine," "feminine," and "ready for sex." Notes in the margins highlight issues and problems of particular concern to either guys or girls, and funny illustrations add to the reader-friendly tone.

Is It a Choice? Answers to the Most Frequently Asked Questions About Gay and Lesbian People, by Eric Marcus.
Published by HarperSanFrancisco.

Like *Go Ask Alice*, this thorough, straightforward, easy-to-read book follows a question and answer format. Marcus, a gay journalist, introduces *Is It a Choice?* with the statement: "There's no such thing as a stupid question." He then goes on to answer everything from "Are you born gay?" to "Who plays the husband and who plays the wife?" to "What's it like to be a gay or lesbian teenager?" to "If you're a teenager and think you're gay or lesbian, what should you do?" The answers are based on interviews with gay men and lesbians and the author's own experiences, as well as scientific, psychological, and historical research.

Interpreting Your Quiz Score

Surprise. It's up to you to decide what your score means. Here's why:

Only you can decide whether you're ready to have sex.

Sure, we could tell you that if you score 15 or above, it's OK to have sex, but that might not be true. Because maybe, as far as you're concerned, it's wrong to have sex outside of marriage. If that's the case, even if you have a truly wonderful relationship with someone you're very attracted to, you shouldn't do it. Since we can't possibly know that about you, we can't really tell you that you're "ready" or "not ready" to have sex just because you got a high score. (However, that high score does tell us that you probably have a pretty good relationship going—congratulations!)

And what if your score was below 10? Perhaps you just met someone and don't know them very well, but you're incredibly attracted to this person and you want to have sex right now. If you're responsible about diseases, birth control, and each others' feelings, then...it's a risk, but maybe you're ready to have sex even if you don't know each other's favorite colors. Again, that's for you to decide, not us.

We hope reading this book has helped you figure out what will make you feel good about your decision to have sex—or not have it—so that you'll be less likely to have regrets later on. If you can think of any other things that teens should know or do before having sex, please send them to us and we'll consider them for the next edition of this book. Send your suggestions to:

The Editors
The Teen Guide to Sex
c/o Youth Communication
224 West 29th Street, 2nd Fl.
New York, NY 10001

Or email: info@youthcomm.org

Index of Questions

5 Things to Ask About Intimacy

5 Things to Ask Your Partner About Sex

5 Things to Ask About Each Other's Bodies

5 Things to Ask About Where, When, and How

5 Things to Ask About Dealing With the Consequences

A Note to Adults

For more than 25 years, Youth Communication has published magazines written by and for teenagers which address the most important issues in their lives. It should come as no surprise that one of the most popular topics is sex. Kids who haven't had sex have questions they want to explore: How do you do it? What does it feel like? How will I know I'm ready? Will I be different afterwards? Kids who have done it have questions too: Why did I do it? Why didn't I use protection? Why don't we feel closer? Why do we feel closer?

What concerned us most was not that so many of the teens we knew were having sex, but that so much of the sex they were having was both joyless and careless. Although we've run a handful of positive stories about teens' sexual experiences over the past three decades (stories about how good it feels or how it brought a couple closer), the vast majority of the stories have been tinged with regret. They are stories about repercussions, from broken hearts to unplanned pregnancies to STDs. They are stories about sex that just wasn't very good—because it was rushed, or with someone the writer didn't know very well or didn't really care about, or because the couple didn't use protection and the writer spent the whole time worrying about catching something.

When we ask the young people who write these stories why they did what they did (Why have sex with someone you don't have feelings for? Why have sex without a condom?), the most common answer is, "It just happened."

Many young (heterosexual) women, in particular, seem to feel that they have little control over their sex lives. Some seem to feel that if they have boyfriend who treats them halfway decently, they owe it to him to have sex even if they don't really want to. Some who want to have sex seem to feel that once they agree to do it, they've given up their right to set any boundaries or make any demands (like "only if we use a condom"). Some just feel too uncomfortable or embarrassed to discuss the things that are on their minds (like "Is there any chance you could have an STD?" or "What would you do if I got pregnant?"). And some—too many—are pressured or forced to have sex when they don't want to.

Guys feel pressure too, of course. They're supposed to want to have sex anytime, anywhere, with anyone. It's not easy for them to say, "We can't, I don't have a condom" or, "Do you want a relationship or just a one-night stand?" And while they can't get pregnant, they can (and do) suffer from STDs and broken hearts.

This is not to say that there are no teens out there choosing to have sex because they really want to, and taking responsible precautions. But we've heard enough teens say that they wish they had waited—until they were more mature, until they were really in love, until they were confident enough to ask for what they really wanted and refuse to do things that made them uncomfortable—to know that too many teens are letting sex happen to them rather than making thoughtful decisions about when, where, with whom, and under what circumstances they should have sex.

So we began a dialogue in our program involving adult and teen staff members—male and female, virgins and non-virgins, straight, gay, bisexual, and transgender. People who had had sex talked about what they wish they had known before doing it, the mistakes they'd made and regrets they had, as well as the times when it felt right and what had made it feel right. People who hadn't had sex yet talked about their questions, their fears, and what they would want their first sexual experience to be like. We also ran essay contests in our magazines, asking teen readers what they thought teens should know or do before having sex, which drew hundreds of responses.

Based on our discussions, the essays and letters submitted by readers, and the dozens of stories about sex that we've published over the years, we came up with scores of questions that teens should ask themselves before having sex—some playful or offbeat, some direct and serious. Our teen writers and adult staff then wrote and rewrote answers to those questions, adding, discarding, and combining questions as we went along. The process was mostly informal and open-ended. But at several stages we asked teens from diverse backgrounds and experiences to read a draft of all the questions and answers developed to that point, prepare written responses, and then spend several hours discussing the material. As we neared the end of the discussion, which had been punctuated by a fair number of comments about bad sexual experiences that the teens had had or heard about, one 18-year-old girl smiled shyly and said, "Now I know why sex with my boyfriend is so enjoyable. I can answer almost all of these questions!"

In this book, we share those questions and explain why knowing the answers will lead to better sexual experiences (or, in many cases, to delayed sexual experiences, as teens realize that the conditions for good sex do not yet exist for them). As the question on page 16 points out, there are good reasons and bad reasons to have sex. People with good reasons have a better chance of having good sex—especially if it's their first time.

Supplementing the Q&A sections of the book are a series of firsthand accounts by teens that detail how they came to have sex (or why they decided not to) and how becoming sexually active has changed their lives—for better and for worse. These forthright, thoughtful accounts cover a wide range of experiences: What it's like to have the guy you've been dating for more than a year dump you after you start having sex or to find out that your dream girl has given you an STD; how a 14-year-old girl can be sure that having sex with her boyfriend was the right decision, while an 18-year-old teen mom can feel that she should have waited.

We want teens to understand that sex isn't something that just happens to them—they have choices. Before making those choices, it makes sense to take the time to think about what they want and what they value and to weigh the risks involved for themselves and their potential partners (and do everything they can to minimize those risks). This book will help.

Who is this book for?

Age: There is a wide range of opinion about what information young people should get about sex and at what age. Please use your judgment in using this book with young people, taking into account their developmental stage and the rules and expectations of your institution, if you are using it in a school, for example.

Here are two things to keep in mind. First, in writing this book, our target audience was any youth who are thinking about becoming sexually active. This could range from age 12 (or even younger) to age 19 or over. Second, we have talked with hundreds of teens about sex. Many teens have said that adults waited too long to have frank and helpful conversations with them about sex. So far, no teen has ever said that adults initiated those conversations too early.

Gender: This book is equally suitable for boys and girls, and can be used in single-sex or mixed groups.

Sexual orientation: This book is designed to address the concerns of teens of any sexual orientation.

Credits

The stories in this book originally appeared in the following Youth Communication publications:

"Womanhood Can Wait," by Nicole Hawkins, *New Youth Connections*, September/October 1998; "I Need a Girl," by Destiny, *New Youth Connections*, May/June 2002; "Why I Hate Sex," by Lenny Jones, *New Youth Connections*, November 1997; "Looking for Love," by Fetima P., *Represent*, May/June, 1998; "Virgin Under Pressure," by Anonymous, *New Youth Connections*, December 2003; "I Wasn't Pressured," by Anonymous, *New Youth Connections*, September/October 1999; "Infatuation With Masturbation," by Tasha, *New Youth Connections*, November 2005; "Learning Without Doing," by Nadishia Forbes, *New Youth Connections*, September/October 1999; "How to Buy a Condom," by Cassaundra Worrell, *New Youth Connections*, December 1987; "My Best Friend Has an STD," by Anonymous, *New Youth Connections*, April 2004; "The Morning After," by Anonymous, *New Youth Connections*, May/June 2002; "What if I'm Pregnant?" by Genevieve Santos, *New Youth Connections*, May/June 2002; "Ready for Mr. Right," by Faleisha Escort, *New Youth Connections*, March 1999; "Nothing Like the Real Thing," by Eric Green, *Represent*, November/December, 2008; "Me and Zarah...Zarah and Everyone Else," by Anonymous, *New Youth Connections*, December, 2001; "Messing Around Is No Match for Love," by Christian Galindo, *New Youth Connections*, May/June 2002; "Younger Girls/Older Guys," by Anonymous, *New Youth Connections*, March 2002; "Looking for Maturity," by Anonymous, *New Youth Connections*, March 2002; "I Paid a High Price for Love," by Anonymous, *New Youth Connections*, November 1996; "Haunted by My Past," by Anonymous, *Represent*, January/February 2007; "Rush to Love," by Jennifer Ramos, *New Youth Connections*, December 2002; "Opening Up to My Girl," by Antwaun Garcia, *Represent*, January/February 2003; "Trusting Him With the Truth," by Anne Ueland, *Represent*, January/February 2000; "Performance Anxiety," by Anonymous, *New Youth Connections*, December 2001; "Love Made Me Carefree...and Careless," by Lenny Jones, *New Youth Connections*, September/October 1999; "Put Yourself Before Sex," by Nicole Hawkins, *New Youth Connections*, September/October 1998; "How I Stopped Giving In," by Anonymous, *New Youth Connections*, September/October 1996; "There's More to Sex Than Sex," by Loretta C., *New Youth Connections*, September/October 1992; "The First Time," by Jasmin Urias, *New Youth Connections*, September/October 1999; "Am I the Father?" by Anonymous, *New Youth Connections*, December 2003; "Abortion Was the Right Choice for Me," by Lakia H., *Represent*, May/June 2001; "My Sex Story," by Anonymous, *New Youth Connections*, March 2003; "A Family to Raise Her," by Jennifer Olensky, *Represent*, May/June 2001; "Teen Mothers Grow Up Fast," by Janice Brooks, *New Youth Connections*, November 1999; "My Boyfriend Lied," by Anonymous, *Represent*, September/October 2006; "Why I Always Use a Condom," by Anonymous, *Strange Brew*, June 1992; "All About Birth Control," by Rasheeda Raji and Kymberly Sheckleford, *New Youth Connections*, December, 2003; "The GYN Exam, Explained," by Madeleine Gordillo, *New Youth Connections*, November 1996.

Acknowledgments

This book was under development at Youth Communication for more than 10 years. During that time dozens of teens and other people provided helpful comments. Thank you to these readers who provided especially thorough comments:

Teens: Reginald Cazeau, Christine Cosme, Cheryl Ann Davis, Christine Gonzalez, Keshia Harrell, Phillip Hodge, Jose Jimenez, Jackie Miller, Jennifer Ramos, Rasheeda Raji, Elizabeth Sanchez, Jessica Santiago, Shannell Walker, and Yen Yam.

Adults: Ruth Bell, Kelsey Fuller, Andy Humm, Craig Schommer, Peggie Schommer, and Susan N. Wilson.

Thanks also to the 2001-02 teen writers at Sex, etc. and the 2002 Teen Advocacy group at Planned Parenthood of New York City.

About
Youth Communication

Youth Communication, founded in 1980, is a nonprofit youth develop-ment program located in New York City whose mission is to teach writ-ing, journalism, and leadership skills. The teenagers we train become writers for our websites and books and for two print magazines: *New Youth Connections*, a general-interest youth magazine, and *Represent*, a magazine by and for young people in foster care.

Each year, up to 100 young people participate in Youth Communication's school-year and summer journalism workshops, where they work under the direction of full-time professional editors. Most are African-American, Latino, or Asian, and many are recent immigrants. The opportunity to reach their peers with accurate portrayals of their lives and important self-help information motivates the young writers to create powerful stories.

Our goal is to run a strong youth development program in which teens produce high quality stories that inform and inspire their peers. Doing so requires us to be sensitive to the complicated lives and emotions of the teen participants while also providing an intellectually rigorous experience. We achieve that goal in the writing/teaching/editing relation-ship, which is the core of our program.

Our teaching and editorial process begins with discussions between adult editors and the teen staff. In those meetings, the teens and the editors work together to identify the most important issues in the teens' lives and to figure out how those issues can be turned into stories that will resonate with teen readers.

Once story topics are chosen, students begin the process of crafting their stories. For a personal story, that means revisiting events in one's past to understand their significance for the future. For a commentary, it means developing a logical and persuasive point of view. For a reported story, it means gathering information through research and interviews. Students look inward and outward as they try to make sense of their experiences and the world around them and find the points of intersection between personal and social concerns. That process can take a few weeks or a few months. Stories frequently go through ten or more drafts as students work under the guidance of their editors, the way any professional writer does.

Many of the students who walk through our doors have uneven skills, as a result of poor education, living under extremely stressful conditions, or coming from homes where English is a second language. Yet, to complete their stories, students must successfully perform a wide range of activities, including writing and rewriting, reading, discussion, reflection, research, interviewing, and typing. They must work as members of a team and they must accept individual responsibility. They learn to provide constructive criticism, and to accept it. They engage in explorations of truthfulness, fairness, and accuracy. They meet deadlines. They must develop the audacity to believe that they have something important to say and the humility to recognize that saying it well is not a process of instant gratification. Rather, it usually requires a long, hard struggle through many discussions and much rewriting.

It would be impossible to teach these skills and dispositions as separate, disconnected topics, like grammar, ethics, or assertiveness. However, we find that students make rapid progress when they are learning skills in the context of an inquiry that is personally significant to them and that will benefit their peers.

When teens publish their stories—in *New Youth Connections* and *Represent*, on the web, and in other publications—they reach tens of thousands of teen and adult readers. Teachers, counselors, social workers, and other adults circulate the stories to young people in their classes and out-of-school youth programs. Adults tell us that teens in their programs—including many who are ordinarily resistant to reading—clamor for the stories. Teen readers report that the stories give them information they can't get anywhere else, and inspire them to reflect on their lives and open lines of communication with adults.

Writers usually participate in our program for one semester, though some stay much longer. Years later, many of them report that working here was a turning point in their lives—that it helped them acquire the confidence and skills that they needed for success in college and careers. Scores of our graduates have overcome tremendous obstacles to become journalists, writers, and novelists. They include National Book Award finalist and MacArthur Fellowship winner Edwidge Danticat, novelist Ernesto Quiñonez, writer Veronica Chambers, and New York Times reporter Rachel Swarns. Hundreds more are working in law, business, and other careers. Many are teachers, principals, and youth workers, and several have started nonprofit youth programs themselves and work as mentors—helping another generation of young people develop their skills and find their voices.

Youth Communication is a nonprofit educational corporation. Contributions are gratefully accepted and are tax deductible to the fullest extent of the law.

To make a contribution, or for information about our publications and programs, including our catalog of over 100 books and curricula for hard-to-reach teens, see www.youthcomm.org.

About the Editors

Andrea Estepa edited *New Youth Connections*, Youth Communication's magazine by and for New York City teens, from 1991 to 1997. Prior to that, she was a reporter for *The Hartford Courant* and the *Los Angeles Times*. In 1997 she was awarded a Revson Fellowship by Columbia University. Estepa has a master's degree from the Graduate School of Journalism at Columbia and a bachelor's degree from Brown University. She is currently finishing her doctorate in history of women and gender from Rutgers University.

Keith Hefner co-founded Youth Communication in 1980 and has directed it ever since. He is the recipient of the Luther P. Jackson Education Award from the New York Association of Black Journalists and a MacArthur Fellowship. He was also a Revson Fellow at Columbia University.

Laura Longhine is the editorial director at Youth Communication. She edited *Represent*, Youth Communication's magazine by and for youth in foster care, for three years, and has written for a variety of publications. She has a BA in English from Tufts University and an MS in Journalism from Columbia University.

Nora McCarthy is a former editor of Youth Communication's two teen magazines: *Represent* and *New Youth Connections*. In 2005, she founded Rise, a nonprofit that trains parents to write about their experiences with the child welfare system. A graduate of the Medill School of Journalism at Northwestern University, Nora has written about youth and child welfare issues for *Newsday*, *City Limits*, and *Child Welfare Watch*.

Rachel Blustain has a BA from Brown University and an MSW from Hunter College School of Social Work. She worked as a journalist for the *Forward*, where she was the Moscow correspondent. At Youth Communication, she was the editor of *New Youth Connections* magazine, and *Represent*. She is currently a social worker.

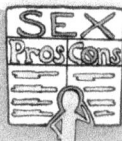

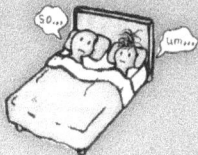

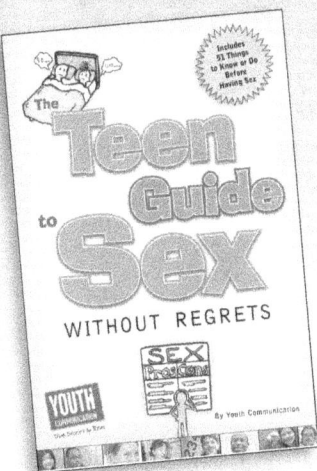

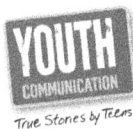

More Helpful Books From Youth Communication

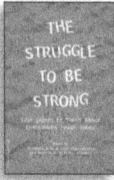

The Struggle to Be Strong: True Stories by Teens About Overcoming Tough Times. Foreword by Veronica Chambers. Help young people identify and build on their own strengths with 30 personal stories about resiliency. (Free Spirit)

Starting With "I": Personal Stories by Teenagers. "Who am I and who do I want to become?" Thirty-five stories examine this question through the lens of race, ethnicity, gender, sexuality, family, and more. Increase this book's value with the free Teacher's Guide, available from youthcomm.org. (Youth Communication)

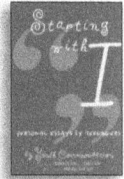

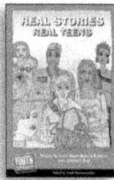

Real Stories, Real Teens. Inspire teens to read and recognize their strengths with this collection of 26 true stories by teens. The young writers describe how they overcame significant challenges and stayed true to themselves. Also includes the first chapters from three novels in the Bluford Series. (Youth Communication)

Out With It: Gay and Straight Teens Write About Homosexuality. Break stereotypes and provide support with this unflinching look at gay life from a teen's perspective. With a focus on urban youth, this book also includes several heterosexual teens' transformative experiences with gay peers. (Youth Communication)

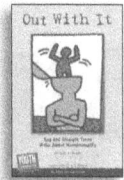

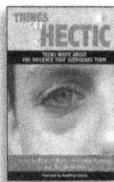

Things Get Hectic: Teens Write About the Violence That Surrounds Them. Violence is commonplace in many teens' lives, be it bullying, gangs, dating, or family relationships. Hear the experiences of victims, perpetrators, and witnesses through more than 50 real-world stories. (Youth Communication)

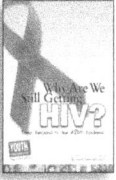

Why Are We Still Getting HIV?: Teens Respond to the AIDS Epidemic Get your teens' attention with true stories by peers who tell how HIV has affected their lives and what teens can do to prevent infection.

Am I Ready?: Girls Write About Sex. Help teen girls make thoughtful choices about sex and relationships by using these stories as a jumping-off point for discussion. (Youth Communication)

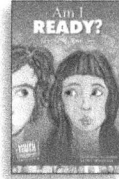

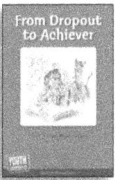

From Dropout to Achiever: Teens Write About School. Help teens overcome the challenges of graduating, which may involve overcoming family problems, bouncing back from a bad semester, or even dropping out for a time. These teens show how they achieve academic success. (Youth Communication)

Why I'm Still a Virgin: Teens Write About Saying No to Sex (Or Wishing They Had). Teens share why they have chosen to abstain from sex, often in the face of extreme peer pressure. They have a variety of reasons—fear, religion, morals, family values, or just a personal sense that they're not ready. (Youth Communication)

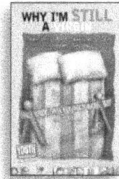

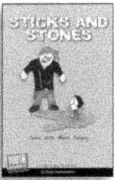

Sticks and Stones: Teens Write About Bullying. Shed light on bullying, as told from the perspectives of the bully, the victim, and the witness. These stories show why bullying occurs, the harm it causes, and how it might be prevented. (Youth Communication)

Through Thick and Thin: Teens Write About Obesity, Eating Disorders, and Self Image. Help teens who struggle with obesity, eating disorders, and body image issues. These stories show the pressures teens face when they are confronted by unrealistic standards for physical appearance, and how emotions can affect the way we eat. (Youth Communication)

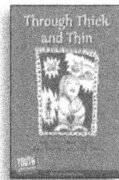

To order these and other books, go to:
www.youthcomm.org
or call 212-279-0708 x115